Pain Medicine
at a Glance

Pain Medicine
at a Glance

BETH B. HOGANS
**The Johns Hopkins School of Medicine and
Veterans Affairs Maryland Health Care System
Baltimore, USA**

WILEY Blackwell

Registered Office(s)
John Wiley & Sons, Inc., 111 River Street, Hoboken, NJ 07030, USA
John Wiley & Sons Ltd, The Atrium, Southern Gate, Chichester, West Sussex, PO19 8SQ, UK

Editorial Office
9600 Garsington Road, Oxford, OX4 2DQ, UK
The Atrium, Southern Gate, Chichester, West Sussex, PO19 8SQ, UK
Boschstr. 12, 69469 Weinheim, Germany
1 Fusionopolis Walk, #07-01 Solaris South Tower, Singapore 138628

For details of our global editorial offices, customer services, and more information about Wiley products visit us at www.wiley.com.

Wiley also publishes its books in a variety of electronic formats and by print-on-demand. Some content that appears in standard print versions of this book may not be available in other formats.

Library of Congress Cataloging-in-Publication Data

Names: Hogans, Beth B. (Beth Brianna), 1964– author.
Title: Pain medicine at a glance / Beth B. Hogans.
Other titles: At a glance series (Oxford, England)
Description: First edition. | Hoboken, NJ : Wiley-Blackwell, 2022. |
    Series: At a glance series | Includes bibliographical references and
    index.
Identifiers: LCCN 2021007910 (print) | LCCN 2021007911 (ebook) | ISBN
    9781118837665 (paperback) | ISBN 9781118837658 (adobe pdf) | ISBN
    9781118837641 (epub)
Subjects: MESH: Pain | Pain Management | Handbook
Classification: LCC RB127 (print) | LCC RB127 (ebook) | NLM WL 39 | DDC
    616/.0472–dc23
LC record available at https://lccn.loc.gov/2021007910
LC ebook record available at https://lccn.loc.gov/2021007911

Cover Design: Wiley
Cover Image: © Science Photo Library - SCIEPRO/Brand X Pictures/Getty Images

Set in 9.5/11.5pt Times by Straive, Pondicherry, India

Printed in Singapore
M087423_250821

Dedicated to E.B. and R.A.

With thanks to my patients and colleagues.

As we meet reality, we must learn to embrace it as a profound set of contingencies in which we are embedded, and whose meaning is unknown.

Polly Young-Eisendrath

The Present Heart

Contents

Preface

Fifteen years in the making, this book was first conceptualized as one of the potential outgrowths from the first-year medical student course in pain at Johns Hopkins assembled by an interprofessional team of pain experts. In the ensuing years, tremendous changes have swept the globe impacting the practice of clinical care: The North American opioid crisis has raised awareness about the perils of medication-based approaches, especially when drugs impacting the reward pathways are used; revisions in healthcare financing, delivery, and education have increased the representation of nurse practitioners and physician assistants in primary care roles; and the gathering of large interprofessional working groups and creation of interprofessional curricula have endeavored to meet to the above needs. This text is responsive to the guidance of the Interprofessional Education Collaborative which recommends that curricula are based on teamwork, shared values, professional roles, and communication, centered on the patient and family, and informed by community and population. The concepts in this book are firmly rooted in the work of the International Association for the Study of Pain but some adaptations are present. The primary target audience of this book is the primary care provider, or nonpain specialist, seeking quick guidance about pain, within the context of an integrated, whole-person approach.

This book springs from my passion for teaching and my profound belief in visual learning. My goal is to change how you think, and feel, about pain – to illuminate the reasons behind pain experience, the events of peripheral nociception, the impacts of pain on the person, and the outlines of how manage pain in the most holistic manner possible, with compassion and concern for best long-term outcomes. With Pain Medicine at a Glance, it is my intention to capture the imagination and attention of each person who happens upon the book, to provide a series of visual mental images that imprint "pain logic" on the mind and aid each reader to approach pain with enthusiasm and interest.

My guiding inspiration for this book was to employ visual learning to change how healthcare providers think about pain. As a young person, I spent many weekends with my grandparents, my grandfather was a naturalist, and my grandmother had grown up on the farm but moved to the city as a teenager to study nursing. They both loved the outdoors but approached it as an opportunity to learn as well as to wonder and enjoy. They had a small collection of guidebooks with exquisite illustrations – trees, mushrooms, wildflowers, seashells, and birds came to life in glorious detail. I loved to gaze at the pictures but was awestruck at how much my grandparents had learned about the world around them and the gentle respect for nature that suffused their approach to exploring that world. Pain Medicine at a Glance is my chance to share the special love and wonder I feel for the human body as a physician and pain scientist. In it, I seek to unlock some fundamental knowledge so that students and colleagues can better understand and respond to this physiological system that functions to protect us, but sometimes causes profound suffering. May this book be a useful guide on your journey to helping others.

Beth B. Hogans
Baltimore, Maryland

Foreword

No North American pain educator today is more highly esteemed than Beth Hogans. Her career has been informed not only by her medical and scientific training as a scientist and neurologist, but also by broad interests in literature and the humanities. Dr. Hogans' early work identified, in a series of landmark studies, deficits and gaps in the medical student curriculum related to pain. Together with colleagues, she inaugurated an innovative course at Johns Hopkins for entering medical students about pain. For over a decade, this course has served as a model for other pain educators. It spans not only conventional biomedical content but also the experiential and social dimensions of pain. As the course has evolved, so have the fields of pain research, education, and policy. Throughout this time, Beth led the charge to more broadly advance clinical competence in pain. Working collaboratively, she created a scholarly journal section dedicated to pain education. Through this, she guided her peers in the field, raising the level of scholarship in pain education and supporting the development of clinician-educators, nationally and internationally, continually seeking to innovate and disseminate academic advances. Central among these advances has been the reaffirmation that pain is a clinically salient subjective experience heavily influenced by social processes such as isolation and stigma that add to suffering.

Advances in educational psychology have been applied by Dr. Hogans and colleagues to render pain education more effective and efficient. The techniques of role-playing, narrative, re-enactment of brief pain, such as BandAid removal, have been incorporated into the course. Beth has had a particular interest in harnessing the neurobiology of learning to optimize pain education, whether through ensuring that experiences are of relatively brief duration so as not to overload students' cognitive capacity, and providing copious illustrations to harness other means to convey packets of knowledge, e.g. text. The practical results of such a sophisticated approach are embodied in *Pain Medicine at a Glance*: focused one- to two-page chapters that convey the essence of a topic or clinical situation in a way that all members of an interprofessional pain care team can quickly absorb and apply. The consistent delivery of linked pieces of knowledge by a single exemplary clinician-educator-scientist – with practical dicta such as watching out for their own safety, or displaying compassion and empathy – conveys what it must be like for a student or fellow to accompany Beth in the clinic or on bedside rounds.

I believe that the magic by which Dr. Hogans' presence and style suffuse this book derives from its being a single-author volume. Those who know Beth or have heard her speak will recognize the prose of the present volume as conveying her voice. Single-author volumes on complex topics (think Bonica, Beecher, Ballas on sickle cell pain, or Selye on stress) are becoming more and more uncommon as fewer and fewer scholars – particularly clinician-scholars – have the breadth of knowledge to single-handedly convey their oeuvre. Two thousand years ago, Horace, the Roman playwright, satirist, and father of literary criticism, in *Ars Poetica* urged writers to choose their subject judiciously, in harmony with their own interests and abilities. That done, "neither elegance of style nor clarity of expression shall desert the [writer] by whom the subject matter is chosen judiciously." Devoting her career to becoming an exemplary clinician-educator, Beth has indeed chosen her subject wisely. Her descriptions of problematic situations and how to manage them (e.g. tapering opioids in a patient reluctant to do so) speak with clinical credibility. This volume is a testament to her mastery of the field of pain, and her own personal approach to interdisciplinary pain education, that call to mind the historical mission statement of a leading Boston hospital: "where science and kindliness unite."

Daniel B. Carr, MD, DABPM, FFPMANZCA (Hon.)
Professor Emeritus, Tufts University School of Medicine, Boston
Founding Director, Tufts Program on Pain Research, Education and Policy
Past President, American Academy of Pain Medicine
Honorary Member, International Association for the Study of Pain.

Acknowledgment

Many thanks to Anne Hunt, James Watson, Vincent Rajan, Samras Johnson, and Avinash Singh, my editors at Wiley. I appreciate their consistent encouragement and sage advice in preparing this manuscript. The work came together with a breathtaking team effort – my vision of communicating the wonders of pain clinical science, so many years in the making, has now arrived. Thank you.

I would like to acknowledge some of my many great teachers in pain: Jim Campbell, the late John W. (Jack) Griffin, Jennifer Haythornthwaite, Lewis Levy, Steven Waxman, George Richerson, Alan Pestronk, David Cornblath, Vinay Chaudhry, Ahmet Hoke, Andrea Corse, Stuart Goldman, Steve McMahon (Mac), Dan Carr, and Mac Gallagher have taught me so much about pain and nociceptive processing. Paul Hoffman, Dick Meyer, and Tom Brushart were among my exemplars of critical scientific reasoning. Judy Watt-Watson, Pat Thomas, Margaret Lloyd, Nancy Hueppchen, Andy Levy, Kyle Davis, Beth Nenortas, Christina Spellman, and Rachel Salas are among my great educational role models. I am deeply grateful to David Yarnitsky, Merav Shor, Antje Barreveld, Michelle Taylor, and Bernie Siaton for professional collaborations and sincere friendship. I have been fortunate to have many wonderful students, but some have brought exceptional effort and talent including Aakash Agarwal, Lina Mezei, Joe Nugent, Alexis Steinberg, Zelda Ghersin, and Kolade Fapohunda. Mr. Tim Foley is an extraordinary and talented administrator, and I am most appreciative of Ms. Tina Moore's heartfelt and able administrative support of my academic career. Les Katzel has supported my advanced career development with grace and wit, and John Sorkin has championed my passion for statistics and applied mathematics in the service of clinical medicine. Justin McArthur has always offered encouragement and fostered my passion for neurology and pain. Shelley List, my dear friend, has served unswervingly as a personal ad hoc editor, consultant, and trusted advisor. My father Donald Hogans was an extraordinarily devoted champion; given his 2-meter stature, from birth, I actually "stood on the shoulders" of a giant. He cheered my efforts to write cogently about pain and to step up to any reasonable opportunity to improve the world. And my children, who have genuinely been my light and joy – so determined, so clever, and so unfailingly kind.

To apportion our days?
But tell us how,
and we shall come to the heart of wisdom.
The Psalm of Moses

Beth B. Hogans
Baltimore, MD

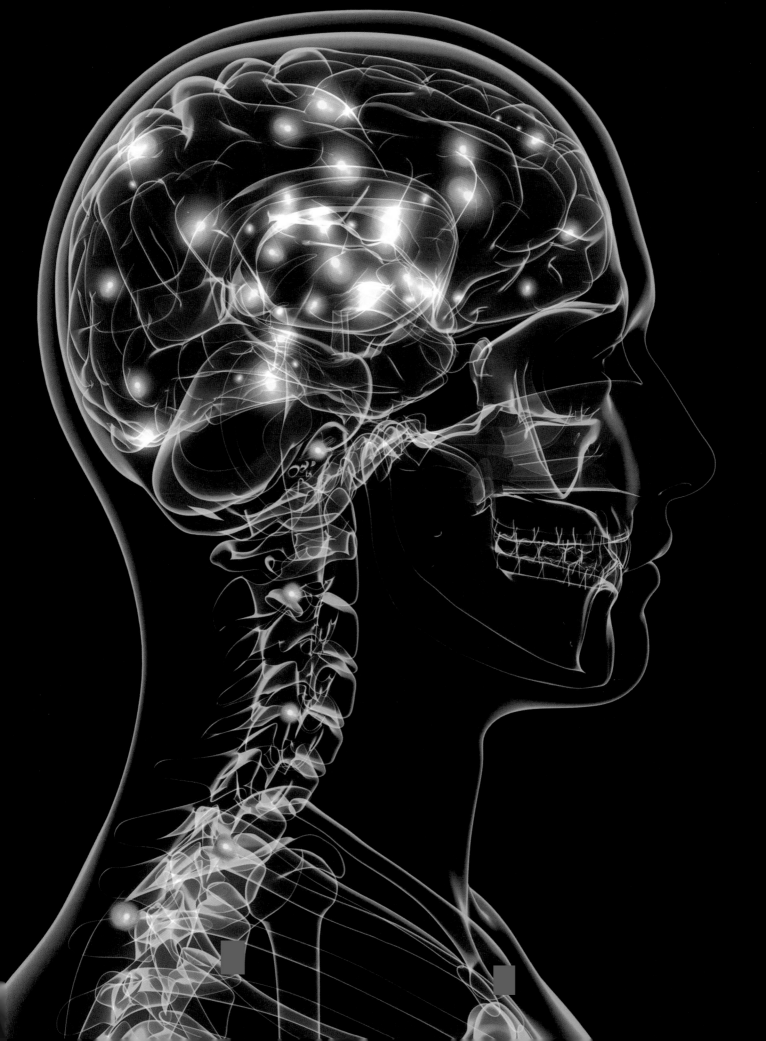

1 What is pain and how do we assess it?

Formally defined as an "unpleasant sensory and emotional experience associated with, or resembling that associated with, actual or potential tissue damage" (Raja et al. 2020), pain has an enormous impact on clinical outcomes. This formal definition captures several important aspects of pain: first, it is **unpleasant**, meaning that most people strongly prefer pain relief to continued pain. Second, pain is a **sensory** AND **emotional** experience, which means that pain has both *sensory-discriminative* qualities, i.e. descriptive features such as burning or stabbing; as well as *unpleasantness*, i.e. aspects that pertain to suffering (Figure 1.1). The unpleasantness of pain profoundly motivates most people to seek relief. The *suffering* associated with pain motivated Epicurean philosophers (300 BCE) to observe in that the height of pleasure is reached with the absence of pain.

Essential to survival, pain normally functions as a warning sign of *damage* to the body. High mortality rates are associated with *painless* myocardial ischemia; patients who cannot perceive a heart attack won't seek medical care until it is too late. At the extreme end of this spectrum are patients born with genetic mutations that eliminate pain sensing, e.g. SCN9A sodium channel defects, these patients are at increased risk for mutilation and death (Cox et al. 2006).

Perhaps the most important aspect of pain the tremendous variability from one person to another, **interindividual variability**, Figure 1.2. Due to diverse biology, genetic, and environmental factors, it is truly not possible to "know another's pain." We must ask people about their pain in order to understand it. In a clinical setting, we call this "**pain assessment**."

Standard basic pain assessment includes assessment of: (i) Quality (burning, sharp, etc.), (ii) Region involved (arm, leg, etc.), (iii) Severity (also pain intensity), (iv) Timing (sudden, slow, waxing/waning), (v) Usually associated symptoms (rashes,

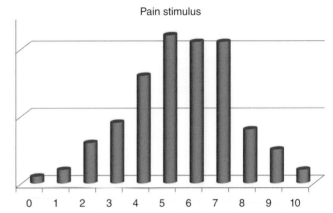

Pain stimulus

Figure 1.2 Interindividual variability in pain showing tremendous variability in healthy individuals exposed to pain stimulus.

Figure 1.3 Standard pain assessment: the pain 'Alphabet'.

> **Q**uality
> **R**egion
> **S**everity
> **T**iming
> "**U**sually associated with"
> "**V**ery much better with"
> "**W**orse with"

vomiting, etc.), (vi) the things which make the pain Very much better (medicines, rest), and (vii) the things which make the pain Worse, Figure 1.3. This information, taken together, enables the clinician to formulate a preliminary **differential diagnosis**. Caring for patients with pain relies on strong basic clinical skills. It is essential to establish a problem list and a working differential diagnosis.

Functional pain assessment includes appraisal of how pain impacts a patient's functioning in daily life. Are they able to: Carry out tasks at home? Work to full capacity? Engage in self-care? Interact with family and friends? Contribute to society normally? Enjoy life? And What is their quality of sleep? How is pain impacting their mood?

Limited pain assessment, at a minimum, focuses on pain severity. Through the use of pain intensity scales, it is possible to rapidly and reproducibly ask patients about pain. Clearly subjective, but highly reproducible, the **numerical rating scale (NRS)** is the preferred pain intensity scale (Figure 1.4). Widely used, it is easy to understand, rapidly explained and scored, does not require literacy, translates well to other languages, and shows robust response properties in clinical practice. Intubated patients can use an NRS presented visually. The NRS is properly referred to as an

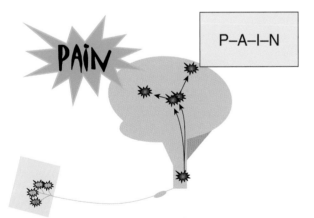

Limbic projections mediate affective content.   Somatosensory projections mediate sensory-discriminative content.

Figure 1.1 Pain has sensory-discriminative and emotional-motivational components.

Pain Medicine at a Glance, First Edition. Beth B. Hogans.
© 2022 John Wiley & Sons Ltd. Published 2022 by John Wiley & Sons Ltd.

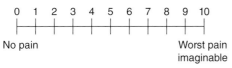

Figure 1.4 The numerical rating scale of pain severity (intensity).

"11-point scale" as 0 and 10 are both included. Changes of less than 2 points on the NRS are generally below the "**minimal clinically significant change**" threshold and not meaningful. Limited pain assessment, focusing on pain severity alone is only appropriate for **ultra-rapid re-assessment** of patients with an established diagnosis. Initial appraisal of a patient with pain should always include the elements of the standard basic assessment, and the functional pain assessment, pain frequently impacts function (Figure 1.5).

Over the years, a number of other pain scales have been used for verbal adults including the 'verbal descriptor scale' (mild/moderate/severe), the visual analog scale (a bar with no tick marks), a 100-point scale, and a pain thermometer. The NRS is currently the most widely preferred scale.

For children, it is important to conduct an **age-appropriate pain assessment**. Infants and pre-verbal children require behavioral pain scales, Chapter 50. For those with communication barriers, cognitive impairments, or dementia, situationally appropriate pain scales are necessary, Chapters 10 and 51.

There are several scales used in research that were designed to assess various aspects of pain. The McGill Pain Questionnaire includes a list of **77 pain descriptors** organized into **20 categories** that are grouped in major domains of sensory, affective and evaluative in nature, and ranging in intensity (Melzack 1975). For example, pain that is pulsatile, ranges from flickering to pounding. Reviewing this instrument can build awareness of the **diverse qualities** of pain descriptors. The Brief Pain Inventory (BPI) is another informative and widely validated pain assessment instrument (Cleeland 2017). The BPI asks about pain in terms of impact on various domains of function: sleep, mood, general activity, relationships with others, etc.; as well as rating pain intensity. Both of these scales are available on the web.

In a nutshell, pain is a major force in life and medicine. It determines many of the choices we make as we navigate potentially hostile and dangerous environments. In the absence of a functioning pain system, we cannot grow to adulthood without repeated traumatic injuries. Conversely, when the pain system goes awry and overamplifies pain, persistent suffering is the result. Through biomedical research and increasing patient-centeredness in clinical care, tremendous strides in understanding and managing the pain

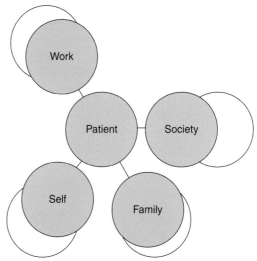

Figure 1.5 Pain interferes with function in multiple domains of daily functioning. A patient may experience varying degrees of impairment.

system are occurring with implications for improved healthcare and patient satisfaction. In this book, you will encounter pain in many different aspects, and learn the beginning steps to assessing and treating pain safely and effectively.

Pain is prevalent and impacts all patient outcomes: learning about pain will improve your clinical performance, enhance your career satisfaction, and increase quality of life for you, and for your patients.

References

Cleeland, C. (2017). Brief pain inventory user guide. https://www.mdanderson.org/documents/Departments-and-Divisions/Symptom-Research/BPI_UserGuide.pdf (accessed 17 December 2017).

Cox, J.J., Reimann, F., Nicholas, A.K. et al. (2006). An SCN9A channelopathy causes congenital inability to experience pain. Nature 444 (7121): 894–898.

Melzack, R. (1975). The McGill pain questionnaire: major properties and scoring methods. Pain 1 (3): 277–299. doi: 10.1016/0304-3959(75)90044-5. PMID: 1235985.

Raja, S.N., Carr, D.B., Cohen, M. et al. (2020). The revised International Association for the Study of Pain definition of pain: concepts, challenges, and compromises. Pain 2020 Sep 1; 161 (9): 1976–1982. doi: 10.1097/j.pain.0000000000001939. PMID: 32694387; PMCID: PMC7680716.

2 Nociceptive processing: How does pain occur?

Nociceptive processing is the processing of pain-related information by the nervous system, occurring at many levels. By understanding how pain is processed in the body, we can better understand patients' pain.

Both **neurons** and **glia** participate in nociceptive processing and responses to nociceptive inputs are shaped by **genetic** and **environmental** factors, explaining the tremendous **variation** in pain experience.

The nociceptive processing system is anatomically and functionally divided into four inter-related components: transduction, transmission, perception, and modulation (Figure 2.1). Normally, nociceptive processing serves to protect an organism. Unfortunately, fidelity in recognizing threats is sometimes lost, and **misdirected activation** results in **aberrant pain sensing** (enhancement or loss). In this respect, the pain system is not unlike the immune system which can manifest disorders of excessive or deficient immunity, both causing substantial harm. Excessive pain, persistent pain, and deficient pain perception are all detrimental to health.

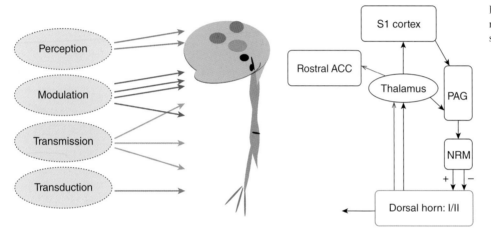

Figure 2.1 Simplified overview of nociceptive processing in the nervous system.

Transduction

Pain perception normally begins with a noxious stimulus. Perhaps a thorn is encountered: nerve endings of thinly myelinated and unmyelinated axons respond. Many decades ago, there was vigorous discussion about the "**labeled line**" **hypothesis**. The idea was that "pain" was encoded by specific nerve fibers and travelled in a dedicated pain system. With molecular biology, we know now that there are a wide variety of "labeled lines" each carrying signals of a particular flavor or nuance (Stucky et al. 2009; Ringkamp et al. 2013). For example, various **transient receptor-potential (TRP) channels** are expressed in sensory neurons responding to high heat, medium heat, low heat, warm, and cold stimuli across the thermal spectrum, similar to the way that rods in the eye respond to different spectral intensities of light (Tominaga et al. 1998; Fernández-Carvajal et al. 2012). Some of these thermal stimuli are clearly encoded as painful, some require co-activation of other sensory afferents to produce a painful percept. Transduction occurs in response to different forms of stimulus, e.g. mechanical, thermal, chemical. Signaling ions enter the primary afferent peripheral nerve termination causing small shifts in membrane potential: the "**graded potential**." If the graded potential shifts the local membrane potential to threshold, action potentials volley into the afferent axon. Altered transduction by nerve endings in the target organ is an important part of inflammatory pain; mediators such as NGF, bradykinin, and protons can sensitize nerve endings, leading non- painful stimuli to produce pain.

Transmission

Nociceptive signals are transmitted as **action potentials** via multiple structures in parallel and series. The primary afferent neuron, with cell body located in the dorsal root ganglion, extends axons peripherally and centrally from the sensory ganglion. Many nociceptive signals are transmitted by small nerve fibers of varying caliber. "First pain," for example, is signaled by **thinly myelinated** a-delta fibers that conduct action potentials at about 20 m/s. This means that an adult leg can be traversed in under 50 ms. So-called "second pain" is signaled by **unmyelinated C fibers** that conduct at 1 m/s and arrive at the spinal cord much later. Both fast and slow signals are transmitted to second order neurons in the spinal dorsal horn. The synapses are principally located about two anatomical levels rostral to the entry of the root into the spinal cord. Lumbar and sacral spinal roots terminate far rostral to the corresponding vertebra, with implications for spinal lesion localization. Cervical roots are much shorter. Altogether, nerves, spinal cord, brain stem, and cortical white matter are all involved in transmission.

Pain Medicine at a Glance, First Edition. Beth B. Hogans.

Perception

The perception of pain is **multidimensional** and occurs in several cortical sites. **S1** and **S2** are associated with the sensory-discriminative features of pain. The earliest activation of cortex in response to pain is in the "S2" sensory-discriminative area (Granovsky et al. 2008). The medial limbic cortex, (**rostral anterior cingulate** cortex) mediates the affective, motivational aspects of pain. Other structures contribute to the impact of pain on motor behavior (**basal ganglia** and **cerebellum**), sympathetic tone (**insula**), and alertness (**periaqueductal gray**) (Liu et al. 2011). It is arguable whether all are properly referred to as "perception" but a better term has not arisen. Perception occurs as a complex temporal and spatial series of events varying with the type, severity, and persistence of pain. Neuropathic pain results in strong activation of affective and motivational centers in the brain. Unfortunately, persistent pain may be associated with brain atrophy (Baliki et al. 2011).

Modulation

Pain modulation occurs at every level of the nervous system including end-organs, peripheral nerve, **spinal dorsal horn** and rostral centers. Key modulation events occur in the dorsal spinal cord where descending fibers, especially from the **nucleus raphe magnocellularis** (NRM) synapse and control the transmission of nociceptive signals from primary afferent neurons onto second order neurons (Figure 2.2). This is an important form of gating which has the potential to constrain "pain from

accessing the CNS." The NRM is situated in the ventral midline at the pontomedullary junction. It contains both "ON" and "OFF" cells. **ON cells** have the capacity to sensitize an animal to noxious stimuli, effectively turning the pain system "on," whereas **OFF cells** have the capacity to decrease the transmission of nociceptive signals from primary to secondary afferent, effectively turning pain sensitivity "off." More recently, a role for non-neuronal cells has been recognized in nociceptive modulation (see Chapter 29).

In summary, pain experience arises from the normative functioning of the nociceptive processing system, a complex subsystem of the nervous system including both neuronal and non-neuronal elements. Understanding the component elements of the pain processing system: transduction, transmission, perception, and modulation, may aid clinicians in thinking about patients with pain, and lead them to develop more effective diagnostic and treatment plans.

References

Baliki, M.N., Schnitzer, T.J., Bauer, W.R., and Apkarian, A.V. (2011). Brain morphological signatures for chronic pain. PLoS One 6 (10): e26010.

Fernández-Carvajal, A., Fernández-Ballester, G., Devesa, I. et al. (2012). New strategies to develop novel pain therapies: addressing thermoreceptors from different points of view. Pharmaceuticals 5 (1): 16–48. https://doi.org/10.3390/ph5010016.

Granovsky, Y., Granot, M., Nir, R.-R., and Yarnitsky, D. 'Correspondence information about the author David Yarnitsky (2008). Objective correlate of subjective pain perception by contact heat-evoked potentials. Journal of Pain 9 (1): 53–63.

Liu, C.C., Franaszczuk, P., Crone, N.E. et al. (2011). Studies of properties of "Pain Networks" as predictors of targets of stimulation for treatment of pain. Frontiers in Integrative Neuroscience 5: 80.

Ringkamp, M., Raja, S., Campbell, J., and Meyer, R. (2013). Peripheral mechanisms of cutaneous nociception. In: Wall and Melzack's Textbook of Pain, 6e (eds. M.M. SB, M. Koltzenburg, I. Tracey and D. Turk). Philadelphia, PA: Elsevier Saunders.

Stucky, C.L., Dubin, A.E., Jeske, N.A. et al. (2009). Roles of transient receptor potential channels in pain. Brain Research Reviews 60 (1): 2–23.

Tominaga, M., Caterina, M.J., Malmberg, A.B. et al. (1998). The cloned capsaicin receptor integrates multiple pain-producing stimuli. Neuron 21 (3): 531–543.

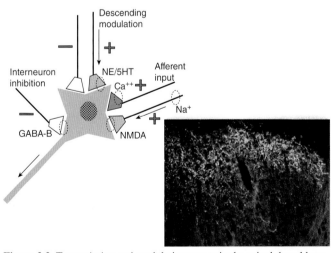

Figure 2.2 Transmission and modulation events in the spinal dorsal horn. Influences on nociceptive processing include: descending inhibition and facilitation, afferent inputs from the periphery and local inhibitory circuits. This is a key site of drug action.

3 What are the major types of pain?

The best approach to understanding and designing effective treatment plans for pain is to view the origins of the problem in terms of **basic pain mechanism**. This is because the pain mechanism has a major impact on: (i) the potential to diagnose a specific condition, (ii) choose an effective treatment, (iii) prognosticate the patient's course in therapy, and (iv) guide the patient in self-management. There are three major *mechanism-based types* of pain: nociceptive, inflammatory, and neuropathic (Figures 3.1 and 3.2).

Nociceptive pain is pain arising from **acute injury**. It is signaled by the **normal functioning** of the nociceptive processing system (Chapter 2). Primary afferents in the various parts of the body are activated by peripheral signaling molecules or direct energy transfer. Currently we know that all of the body is innervated

by afferents with some exceptions: the nucleus pulposus of the vertebral disc, the brain parenchyma, and cartilage. Signaling molecules involved in nociception include: protons, bradykinin, histamine, acetylcholine and others (Ringkamp et al. 2013). Direct energy transfer can occur from pressure-type stimuli, thermal stimuli (hot and cold), or electric shock. A specific nociceptive stimulus may be sensed by multiple primary afferents, as there is no one afferent that is exclusively responsible for pain. Thermal stimuli are sensed by multiple fiber types, for example when touching a hot stove, there is "**first pain**" that provokes an immediate withdrawal response, mediated by Aδ fibers, and "**second pain**" mediated by C fibers that behaviorally reinforce avoidance of damaging stimuli. Nociceptive pain intensity is highly variable depending on personal and contextual factors. Nociceptive pain can be highly responsive to treatments; ideal treatment varies with the intensity, focality, and cause of the pain. In general, mild-to-moderate nociceptive pain responds well to over-the-counter analgesics, e.g. NSAIDs, acetaminophen; severe nociceptive pain may require opioids or special management strategies such as nerve blocks. Nociceptive pain has a good prognosis, but evidence indicates that very strong nociceptive stimuli may predispose patients to chronic pain.

Inflammatory pain is established by exposure to inflammatory signaling molecules and includes pain in response to normally non-painful stimuli. A classic example of this is osteoarthritis: at first, normal walking activity is uncomfortable; later with continued disease, unbearable. Common examples include sunburn, in which light touch fibers are recruited to signal pain making a bag strap intolerable, and ingrown toenails which can make the pressure of a comfortable shoe excruciating. In inflammatory pain, the primary afferents in the body undergo sensitization by inflammatory signaling molecules, including: Nerve Growth Factor (NGF), Tumor Necrosis Factor-alpha (TNFα) Interleukin 6 (IL6), bradykinin, protons, and other substances (Ringkamp et al. 2013). The sensitization of the nerve endings results in long-lasting changes in afferent signaling, termed "**phenotypic switching**." Potentially reversible, the phenotypic switch means that the afferents formerly responsible for nonpainful sensations now signal pain. This is how the pressure of a bag strap or shoe becomes uncomfortable once inflammatory pain signaling is activated. If peripheral inflammation resolves, this increased pain signaling may be reversible. In other situations, such as osteoarthritis, inflammation persists and the pain continues. Inflammatory pain may respond to NSAIDs or corticosteroids, however it is also important to address the origins of inflammatory pain. Specific "**disease-modifying**" therapies include physical therapy, disease-modifying drugs, ergonomic adaptations, or surgery.

Neuropathic pain arises from disease, damage, or **dysfunction** of the nervous system. There are many nervous system conditions manifesting pain including multiple sclerosis, post-herpetic neuralgia, myelopathy, nerve root compression, and peripheral neuropathy.

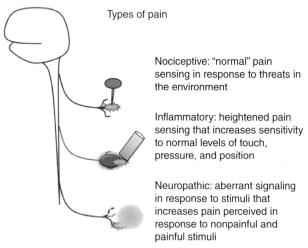

Types of pain

Nociceptive: "normal" pain sensing in response to threats in the environment

Inflammatory: heightened pain sensing that increases sensitivity to normal levels of touch, pressure, and position

Neuropathic: aberrant signaling in response to stimuli that increases pain perceived in response to nonpainful and painful stimuli

Figure 3.1 The basic mechanisms of pain.

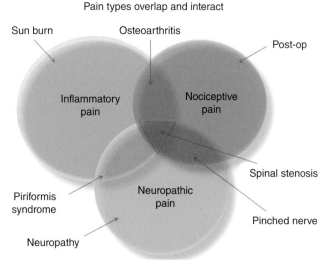

Figure 3.2 How basic pain mechanisms interact.

Pain Medicine at a Glance, First Edition. Beth B. Hogans.

In these cases, pain is driven by **abnormal signaling** arising from the pain-sensing system itself (Devor 2013). This pain can be difficult to treat if the underlying abnormality is not rectifiable. Neuropathic pain is not highly responsive to NSAIDs, and generally prescription medications are required. Multiple treatment options are available. Pain-active anticonvulsants such as gabapentin or pregabalin, or pain-active anti-depressants, such as amitriptyline or duloxetine can provide relief, Chapter 19. Although these **neuromodulating medications** are not universally effective, substantial pain relief may follow when careful attention is applied to titrating medication and addressing the underlying condition. In neuropathic pain, disease modifying therapies are especially valuable. Some forms of neuropathic pain are treatment resistant.

The presence of abnormal pain responses during clinical examination aid in distinguishing nociceptive, inflammatory, and neuropathic pain. Abnormal pain signaling is recognized by the presence of allodynia or hyperalgesia. To explain these terms, it's necessary to introduce the stimulus-response curve. Pain is systematically assessed in clinical and pre-clinical trials using a **stimulus response curve**, this is a graph that represents a person's rating of sensory intensity (pain) in response to a certain stimulus (Figure 3.3). Imagine touching a metal surface of a certain temperature. At room temperature, there is no pain. As the temperature rises, at some point there is a twinge of pain, this is the **pain threshold**. As temperature increases further, pain ratings increase, usually forming an S-shaped curve: at high temperatures the pain ratings are already 10 and further increases don't result in more pain. With neuropathic or inflammatory pain, a person will often feel pain at lower temperatures. The experience of pain in response to a normally non-painful stimulus is called: **allodynia**. This same person may feel more pain in response to stimuli that were previously painful, this is called **hyperalgesia** (see Glossary).

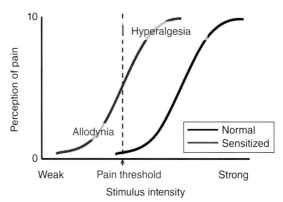

Figure 3.3 Stimulus response curve: normal and abnormal pain perception.

In summary, a mechanism-based classification of pain organizes the clinical approach to the patient with pain and is effective for understanding symptoms, and ultimately planning a diagnostic work up, devising a successful treatment plan, and guiding the patient to effective self-management.

References

Devor, M. (2013). Neuropathic pain: pathophysiological response of nerves to injury. Chapter 61. In: Wall and Melzack's Textbook of Pain, 6e (eds. S.B. McMahon, M. Koltzenburg, I. Tracey and D. Turk). Philadelphia, PA: Elsevier Saunders.

Ringkamp, M., Raja, S., Campbell, J., and Meyer, R. (2013). Peripheral mechanisms of cutaneous nociception. In: Wall and Melzack's Textbook of Pain, 6e (eds. M.M. SB, M. Koltzenburg, I. Tracey and D. Turk). Philadelphia, PA: Elsevier Saunders.

Pain is remarkably prevalent. It is present, at this moment, in millions across the globe. The specifics depend on factors including age, sex, ethnicity, and circumstance, but high pain prevalence is universal (Figure 4.1). In the U.S., data showed 116 million Americans, over one in three, experiencing pain: whether acute procedural pain, trauma, cancer, headache, low back pain, or other pain conditions (IOM 2011). Remarkably, a vast amount of pain is avoided: today millions of surgical procedures annually are performed with **managed pain** due to advances in surgical pain management and medication access worldwide (Chapter 30). Unfortunately, huge challenges persist in pain management as millions experience **limited healthcare access** and others struggle against chronic pain-associated conditions. Here, we explore the challenges.

The common causes of pain are well established and include: headache, low back pain, osteoarthritis, trauma, neuropathy, cancer, and HIV/AIDs primarily (Murphy et al. 2017). Some less common chronic pain conditions, such as CRPS and fibromyalgia, have particularly high healthcare utilization often leading clinicians to overestimate the relevance for education, are described elsewhere (Chapter 45).

Headache is highly prevalent worldwide with nearly half (47%) experiencing headaches at least annually. Most headaches are tension type headaches, 40% experience these. Migraines are less common but more disabling; women more affected than men with global lifetime prevalence (F : M) 22% : 10% and current prevalence 14% : 6% (Stovner et al. 2007). Low back pain is highly prevalent in many countries with 30–40% of adults reporting "current" back pain. **Osteoarthritis** is highly prevalent in older adults with 30% experiencing disabling pain due to arthritis, knee osteoarthritis has been noted as the most common cause of pain-related impairment globally. **Trauma**-related pain, including that related to musculoskeletal injuries is a universal phenomenon with extremely high life-time prevalence, the extent of impairment from work due to musculoskeletal trauma (including back and sprain injuries) exceeds all other causes. **Neuropathy** is prevalent in older adults with 20% over age 75 impacted. Cancer pain is a global burden with 50% of advanced cancer patients reporting pain, access to pain medication is a major determinant in cancer-related

suffering. HIV/AIDS is associated with pain. Recognizing pain cause or basic mechanism is important in clinical practice as the choice of treatment depends on the source of pain and the potential risks of treatment vary with disease context.

Pain prevalence increases with **age** with 50% of older adults experiencing chronic pain. Much of this pain is due to **degenerative joint disease**: lumbosacral DJD, knee and hip osteoarthritis. Peripheral neuropathy increases with age. **Shingles**, a painful eruption of herpes zoster, can cause post-herpetic neuralgia. The incidence of shingles is reduced by 50% with vaccination, CDC recommends vaccination for those age 60 and over.

Certain populations are especially prone to chronic pain, **veterans**, those of lower socioeconomic status, and former athletes. Patients with **cancer** are very likely to experience inadequately controlled pain.

The prevalence of pain varies somewhat between ethnic groups in the United States. Although pain thresholds (minimum detectable pain) are similar across **ethnic groups**, Caucasians generally demonstrate higher experimental pain tolerance than do African Americans, Hispanic, and Asian populations, the reasons are unknown (Kim et al. 2017). Important **disparities** in access to care and impacts on clinical decision-making influence outcomes. These factors generally contribute to higher levels of untreated pain in minority populations (Campbell and Edwards 2012). There is no evidence that people of color experience less pain and proper pain assessment is essential for all patients.

Low socioeconomic status has a negative impact on pain outcomes and predicts a higher prevalence of pain in a population. Many factors may contribute to this especially physical work demands for patients with lower educational attainment and poor access to prompt and effective healthcare. For example, pharmacies located zip codes with lower incomes are less likely to stock opioid medications meaning that patients with cancer and other serious pain-associated conditions cannot obtain WHO essential medications in their own neighborhoods (Green et al. 2005).

There are important, somewhat subtle, differences between how men and women respond to noxious stimuli in the laboratory,

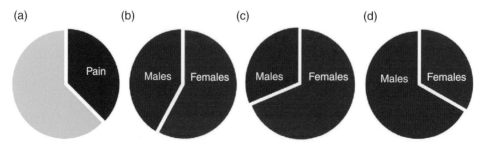

Figure 4.1 (a) Pain is highly prevalent, present in about 38% of the population. (b) Pain overall demonstrates some female preponderance. (c) Migraine, a common headache condition shows female preponderance, 2 : 1, female : male. (d) Cluster headache has a 2 : 1 male preponderance but is much less prevalent (0.1% lifetime prevalence for cluster headache; 14% lifetime prevalence for migraine).

Pain Medicine at a Glance, First Edition. Beth B. Hogans.

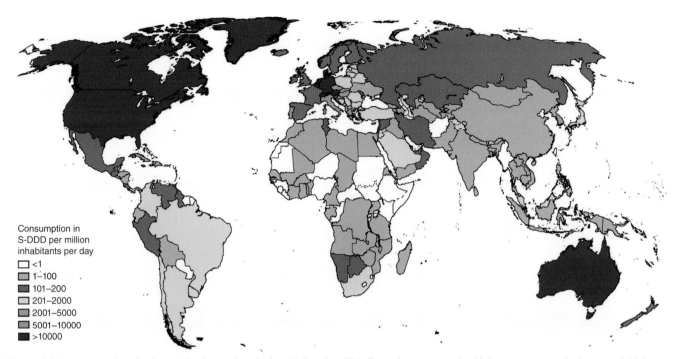

Consumption in
S-DDD per million
inhabitants per day

☐ <1
☐ 1–100
■ 101–200
☐ 201–2000
☐ 2001–5000
☐ 5001–10000
■ >10000

Figure 4.2 Access to pain-relieving medication varies widely with location. This figure demonstrates that high-resource countries have much higher opioid consumption that low-resource countries. Source: Berterame et al. (2016). © 2016, Elsevier.

but similarities abound. In general, men and women respond to pain similarly and the differences between men and women are dwarfed by the interindividual variability in pain sensitivity that we don't yet have explanations for. Nonetheless women on average experience more pain than men. There are important **sex differences** in the prevalence in pain–associated conditions: migraines are much more prevalent in females and cluster headaches much more prevalent in males. There are also **sex-specific pain conditions** such as dysmenorrhea, endometriosis, and testicular torsion.

Pain is an important cause of work-related disability and being engaged in **litigation** or a workman's compensation claim has a negative impact on pain outcomes. Patients may not be conscious of secondary gain however pain persists when there is a matter pending legal resolution.

Finally, **access to care** is a major cause of persistent suffering. Over-reliance on opioids has led to a backlash against assessing pain. In the U.S., opioids cause more **overdose deaths** than any other medication, in other countries, it is impossible to access opioids when clearly appropriate (Figure 4.2). Access to essential medicines, especially opioids is severely restricted in most countries globally so that countries with highest rates of opioid utilization report per capita consumption of 10 000 times more opioids than countries with the lowest rates. WHO estimates that 4.8 million people with cancer die in pain each year without medicine. Globally, millions are dying without relief from pain, there is a pain management crisis of epic proportions.

References

Berterame, S., Erthal, J., Thomas, J. et al. (2016). Use of and barriers to access to opioid analgesics: a worldwide, regional, and national study. The Lancet 387 (10028): 1644–1656. http://www.thelancet.com/cms/attachment/2053462746/2060237771/gr2_lrg.jpg.

Campbell, C.M. and Edwards, R.R. (2012). Ethnic differences in pain and pain management. Pain Management 2 (3): 219–230.

Green, C.R., Ndao-Brumblay, S.K., West, B., and Washington, T. (2005). Differences in prescription opioid analgesic availability: comparing minority and white pharmacies across Michigan. Journal of Pain 6 (10): 689–699. https://doi.org/10.1016/j.jpain.2005.06.002. PMID: 16202962.

Institute of Medicine (US) Committee on Advancing Pain Research, Care, and Education (2011). Relieving Pain in America: A Blueprint for Transforming Prevention, Care, Education, and Research. Washington, DC: National Academies Press.

Kim, H., Yang, G.S., Greenspan, J.D. et al. (2017). Racial and ethnic differences in experimental pain sensitivity: systematic review and meta-analysis. Pain 158: 194–211.

Murphy, K., Han, J.L., Yang, S. et al. (2017). Prevalence of specific types of pain diagnoses in a sample of United States adults. Pain Physician 20: E257–E268.

Stovner, L.J., Hagen, K., Jensen, R. et al. (2007). The global burden of headache: a documentation of headache prevalence and disability worldwide. Cephalalgia 27: 193–210.

5 Pain and ethical practice: How do we resolve dilemmas in pain care?

Modern healthcare ethics stands on four pillars: beneficence, non-maleficence, autonomy, and distributive justice (Beauchamp and Childress 2013; Figures 5.1 and 5.2). Beyond this, an exemplary career in pain-competent healthcare is guided by high levels of compassion, interpersonal insight, resilience, and self-regulation. Every day in pain care, these ideals are tested and tempered. As noted by Giordano (2006) "there is a **core philosophy** of medicine that reflects the intellectual and moral quality of the **healing relationship**". The same is true in nursing, pharmacy, dentistry, physical therapy, social work, clinical psychology, and all health professions. Pain-focused care is rich and fulfilling when actuating the ethical virtues through compassionate connections with patients and others in a joint effort to relieve pain.

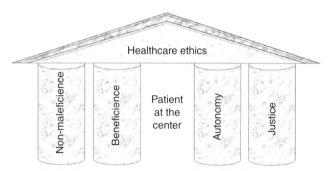

Figure 5.1 Healthcare ethics rests on the "four pillars."

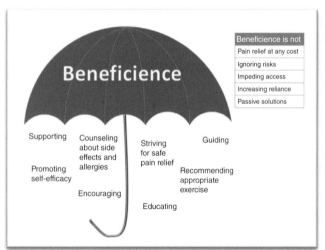

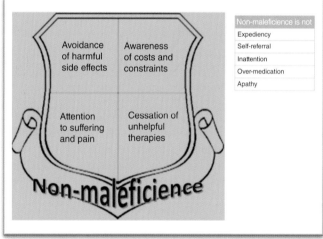

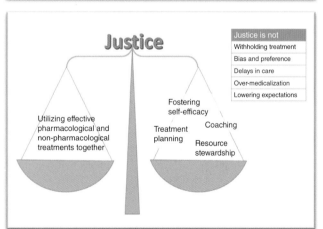

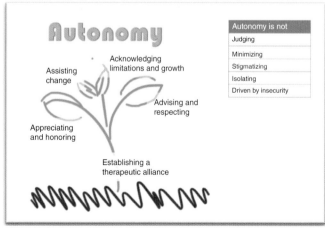

Figure 5.2 Each of the four pillars has distinctive aspects that shape ethical decision-making.

Pain Medicine at a Glance, First Edition. Beth B. Hogans.

Beneficence

Pain care presents frequent opportunities to practice beneficence. In pain care, the overarching goal is the relief of pain, but parallel goals include the **improvement of function** and **quality of life**. In restoring the patient's **confidence** in their ability to manage chronic pain or in alleviating acute pain, there is tremendous beneficence. By learning pain care, whether studying a drug dose, route, and potential interactions; in exploring the mechanisms of focal pain, or in learning how to **support** patients emotionally, we gain an opportunity to help people in the most direct manner: applying our clinical competence to relieve pain and improve lives.

Non-maleficence

The principle of non-maleficence or "doing no harm" has immediate application in pain care where both "not treating" and "treating" have the capacity to harm a patient. For many years, pain was viewed as entirely subjective and not quantifiable, all too often quickly dismissed. No longer; the bygone solution of ignoring or minimizing pain is soundly rejected in modern civilized society. With the advent of functional MRI, we know that pain activates numerous brain centers, including those associated with **suffering**. Medicolegal case law has concluded that **ignoring** a patient with pain, particularly a dying, incapacitated patient, is **inhumane**. The Joint Commission has determined that **pain must be assessed**, safely treated, and re-assessed for relief (Baker 2017).

Another aspect of non-maleficence focuses on safety in implementing a pain treatment plan. **The Joint Commission** recommends that patients treated with opioids be assessed and monitored for **respiratory compromise** (Joint Commission 2012). The assessment of patients for the risks of potential **opioid abuse or misuse** is also part of non-maleficence. Opioids can be safely tapered without direct risk of mortality, but almost all patients find that withdrawal from opioids is painful and excruciatingly difficult, some attempt suicide. Thus, opioid tapering after chronic therapy is often a slow, incremental process (Chapter 49). Finally, we now know that prolonged opioid therapy lowers pain threshold and tolerance potentially worsening pain; the use of opioids for chronic pain should be approached with abundant caution (Chapter 48).

Autonomy

The principle of autonomy is critically important in pain care for both the provider and the patient. It is easy to fall into a pattern of issuing instructions to patients in the belief that this is time efficient. This does not respect a patient's autonomy and may not result in a treatment plan that respects the patient's inclinations and healthcare beliefs. **Motivational interviewing** and **shared decision-making** bring autonomy appropriately into the pain-focused clinical encounter (Chapter 14).

Distributive Justice

The practice of pain care is a continual, pragmatic study of distributive justice. This is because pain medications are viewed as expedient, providing inexpensive pain relief albeit producing cognitive dysfunction, constipation, sedation, abuse risks, and other side effects. In counterpoise with medication risks and benefits, is the substantive **investment of time, energy, and money** required to implement most non-pharmacological strategies. It is a principle of distributive justice that patients should not be exposed to more medical risk than necessary while balancing the costs to society. Why do we still prescribe potentially harmful pain medications when a short course of physical or cognitive therapy would be equally efficacious?

Medical tradition teaches that there were two Pillars at Delphi inscribed with simple but indispensable guidance: **Know thyself**, and **Know thy limits**. All too often, we find ourselves stretching to meet the demands of our patients for better, faster, and less expensive solutions. We may be tempted to perform procedures that we don't know well or try treatments that we don't completely understand. While it is laudable to relieve pain as expeditiously as possible, **safety** is always the first concern. Clinical practice should never overstep the scope of training. Perform a procedure or prescribe a treatment only if you are (i) can perform it with technical proficiency, and (ii) can manage the complications, common and less so. If not trained to recognize and manage the complications of any therapy, interventional, opioid-based, or even NSAIDs, one must refrain from intervening. Unfortunately, not treating pain also carries burdens: patients can despair of improved circumstances. There are many pain clinics and always more options for treatment of pain, **do not destroy hope**. Provide a referral if you cannot act. It is ethical to sustain a patient's hope that pain relief or at least **pain mitigation is a reasonable goal**.

Finally, pain care offers opportunities to work with patients to advance a sense **of self-efficacy** and **personal accomplishment**. The best outcome is engaging with a patient to identify appealing lifestyle changes and active non-pharmacological steps that correct a long-standing pain condition. The opportunity to celebrate these victories with our patients is the true reward of the committed and ethical practice of pain care.

References

Baker, D. (2017). The Joint Commission's Pain Standards: Origins and Evolution. Oak Brook, IL: The Joint Commission.

Beauchamp, T. and Childress, J. (2013). Principles of Biomedical Ethics, 7e. New York: Oxford University Press.

Giordano, J. (2006). Moral agency in pain medicine: philosophy, practice and virtue. Pain Physician 9 (1): 41–46.

Joint Commission (2012). Safe use of opioids in hospitals. The Joint Commission Sentinel Event Alert 49: 1–5.

Perhaps the biggest challenge in pain care is recognizing a pain problem when it presents in a manner that is **atypical**. Because common pain-associated conditions sometimes present in atypical ways and uncommon pain-associated conditions drive surprisingly more healthcare utilization than might otherwise reflect their prevalence, diagnostic challenges in pain medicine are not uncommon.

Pattern recognition is a diagnostic method commonly employed by experts, for this reason, and because pain-conditions often have characteristic "patterns," it is very helpful to learn some of the major pain patterns (Figure 6.1). Some are "referred pain patterns." A referral pattern is the perception of pain in one part of the body in response to nociceptive signaling in another part. **Referred pain** characteristically results in pain being perceived in an unharmed part of the body. This can present a diagnostic challenge. A classic example is cardiac pain referring to the left arm or jaw. Another

classic pattern is the association of foot, ankle, or leg pain with disease of the lumbar spine. This may be unknown to the public but should be known to healthcare providers. What is less well appreciated is that each major system in the body, including viscera, muscles, bones, as well as nerves, has a characteristic referral pattern. Other classic examples include the referral of pancreatic pain to the mid-back; and renal pain to the flank or scrotum. Intriguingly, esophageal pain is generally well localized, whereas injury to the uterine cervix produces diffuse pelvic pain. Collectively, the referral patterns of pain perceived from visceral ailments is called the "**viscerotome**." Less well known are the patterns of **myotomes** (muscle pain-referral patterns) and **sclerotomes** (bone pain-referral patterns) (Bähr and Frotscher 1998). Thus, an important challenge in pain medicine is recognizing the diverse presentations of pain-associated conditions. Often so-called "non-

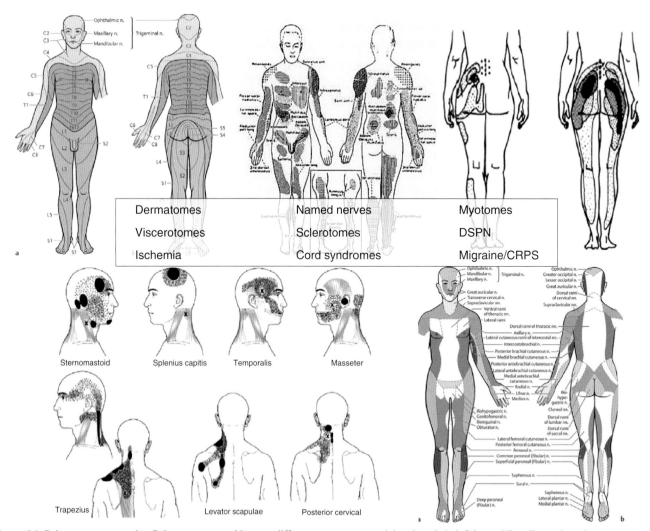

Figure 6.1 Pain patterns, examples. Pain can present with many different patterns, recognizing these is helpful to guiding diagnosis and treatment.

Pain Medicine at a Glance, First Edition. Beth B. Hogans.

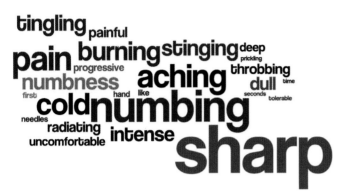

Figure 6.2 Qualities of pain, examples.

anatomical" pain has a biological basis; it simply has not been recognized by the provider. The pictures in Figure 6.1, illustrate some examples of different, anatomical, pain patterns: **dermatomes**, viscerotomes, myotomes, sclerotomes, **diffuse neuropathy**, and **named nerve patterns**. But this catalogue of pain patterns is not exhaustive: still other patterns will be seen with conditions of vascular ischemia or specific pain syndromes such as migraine and chronic regional pain syndrome. Finally, local space occupying lesions can produce bizarre patterns of pain perception, as can neuropathic diseases like multiple sclerosis, transverse myelitis, chronic regional pain syndrome (CPRS), and peripheral neuropathy.

Another critical challenge in pain is: what the pain feels like, known as **qualitative features** or internal experience (Figure 6.2). In this respect, neuropathic pain is the great imitator of modern pain medicine. It is possible for an injured nerve to reproduce a wide variety of ordinary perceptions: burning, cold, and stabbing, as well as produce sensations that are completely bizarre: searing cold, painful numbness, swollen dullness, tingling cascades running down the back, crawling "ants" underneath the skin, and shocking pain so strong it causes the leg to buckle. All of these sensations may arise as the result of nerve damage or dysfunction in a person who, though perhaps **somatically-focused**, is not otherwise prone to thought disorders or delusions. The distress that a person experiences in trying to describe these troubling sensations, or obtain validation within the context of the medical model, is quite real and reasonable.

The **temporal course** of pain is another major challenge in bridging the gap between patient and provider. Sometimes, a person seems to take "too long" to recover from a procedure or trauma. Other times pain seems to flair when **stress** levels are elevated. At times, we risk labeling a stressed "slow healer" as a person with "chronic pain." Other times, there is an **unrecognized trigger** which prompts pain to come and go. One potential cause of profound, intermittent, low back pain is spondylolisthesis. In this disorder, there is an instability of one or more vertebrae. The "typical" experience is terrific pain after arising from being seated on a low support, sometimes getting up from a toilet is the culprit and the patient may be embarrassed. The chronically traumatized disc can become super-sensitized through the ingrowth of pain-

atypical (Stefanakis et al. 2012). Skilled physical therapy, chiropractic, analgesia and core muscle strengthening can help reduce minor to moderate spondylolistheses, more severe instabilities may require surgery. Visceral pain-associated syndromes, e.g. pancreatic, inflammatory bowel disease, and cystitis, are also characterized by a waxing and waning course.

A final challenge is the need to access reliable **unbiased information** about pain medicine diagnoses and treatments. Typically, little time is spent in clinical training on pain. As of 2009, most US medical schools taught only four hours of pain content over four years, this despite the fact that nearly half of patients presenting for medical care have pain of one form or another (Mezei et al. 2011). Not infrequently, providers have trouble determining what's wrong with a "pain patient," because they were not adequately taught to recognize the problem the patient is describing. Exceptions are that osteopathic medical and physical therapy schools offer **advanced training** in musculoskeletal disorders and fellowship pain training is often excellent but may be focused on procedural management (Watt-Watson et al. 2009). For many, collaborative interprofessional care is essential. Reliable resources include Biomed plus for patient-oriented information, UpToDate online, or any of the standard textbooks of pain medicine (Fishman et al. 2009; McMahon et al. 2013; Warfield et al. 2016). Neuromuscular conditions are well characterized online (Pestronk 2017). In short, it is important to learn about common pain-associated conditions and create a differential diagnosis to guide evaluation and treatment strategies.

References

Bähr, M. and Frotscher, M. (1998). Duus' Topical Diagnosis in Neurology: Anatomy, Physiology, Signs, Symptoms, 5e. Stuttgart, New York: Thieme.

Fishman, S.M., Ballantyne, J.C., and Rathmell, J.P. (2009). Bonica's Management of Pain (Fishman, Bonica's Pain Management), 4e. Philadelphia: LWW.

McMahon, S., Koltzenburg, M., Tracey, I., and Turk, D. (eds.) (2013). Wall and Melzack's Textbook of Pain, 6e. Philadelphia, PA: Elsevier Saunders.

Mezei, L., Murinson, B.B., and Johns Hopkins Pain Curriculum Development Team (2011). Pain education in North American medical schools. The Journal of Pain 12 (12): 1199–1208.

Pestronk A (2017) (Ed.). Washington University St. Louis Neuromuscular Disease Center. http://neuromuscular.wustl.edu/ (accessed 18 December 2017).

Stefanakis, M., Al-Abbasi, M., Harding, I. et al. (2012). Annulus fissures are mechanically and chemically conducive to the ingrowth of nerves and blood vessels. Spine 37 (22): 1883–1891.

Warfield, C.A., Bajwa, Z.H., and Wootton, R.J. (2016). Principles and Practice of Pain Medicine, 3e. New York: McGraw-Hill Education/Medical.

Watt-Watson, J., McGillion, M., Hunter, J. et al. (2009). A survey of prelicensure pain curricula in health science faculties in Canadian universities. Pain Research & Management 14 (6): 439–444.

7 Cognitive factors that influence pain

There are many cognitive influences on pain; some of these lessen pain while others increase it. Several cognitive influences are modifiable and have clinical utility in treating pain. Selected cognitive influences on pain are outlined here.

Cognitive influences that increase pain:

Catastrophizing. Catastrophizing describes maladaptive cognitive patterns in response to challenges, especially: imagining a symptom means something ominous (**magnification**), focusing on a problem (**rumination**), and feeling unable to resolve a problem (**helplessness**). Catastrophizing about pain can **amplify pain** intensity and suffering and is associated with poorer long-term outcomes (Quartana et al. 2009). Originally conceptualized by Ellis, catastrophizing has had a great impact on pain research however, large-scale studies are generally needed to show statistical significance. Clinically, effects of catastrophizing on pain are moderate. Cognitive behavioral therapy can help patients shift negative cognitions and replace defeating "self-talk" with more positive messages, it is not known whether single interventions are effective, or whether physicians can administer brief interventions (Turk 2003). For patients with chronic pain who catastrophize, clinical psychological evaluation is indicated.

Anxiety. Anxiety facilitates pain perception. The mechanisms of this are not fully established but one study induced acute pain-associated anxiety which produced increased experimental pain (Rainville et al. 2005). Chronic anxiety is also associated with increased pain in a clinical setting. It is important for healthcare environments to reduce anxiety where possible and ideally providers will create therapeutic relationships sensitive to patients' anxieties. Measures including: reduced jargon, shared decision-making, and utilizing web interfaces and videos to explain procedures in advance can help reduce anxieties. When anxiety is excessive, it is treated with medication and psychotherapy.

Anger. Anger can increase pain. One study of pain-related emotions used hypnotic suggestion to modulate the mood of normal volunteers while pain was tested. In those patients for whom anger was induced, there was a significant increase in perceived pain intensity as well as pain-associated unpleasantness. Anger also has important effects in a clinical setting but the relationship between pain and anger is complex. Studies of patients with low back pain have indicated that the suppression of anger expression increased pain and pain behaviors (Burns et al. 2008). Generally, negative emotions heighten pain while positive emotions reduce pain (Yarns et al. 2020).

Low self-efficacy. Low self-efficacy is when a person feels that they can do little to improve their situation. A related concept is called the "external locus of control." Someone with an external locus of control will feel that their situation is controlled by factors outside themselves. This is contrasted to having an internal locus of control which is when a person feels that they can control their lives and engage in activities that will have a beneficial effect. Patients with internal locus of control have better health-related outcomes. Physicians can foster self-efficacy using motivational interviewing techniques: "What are some small steps you could take to start getting control over your pain?." Many pain self-management strategies require patients to take active steps, e.g., hotpacks, ice, meditation, and pacing require a commitment from patients.

Factors that decrease pain:

Empathetic others. The presence of an empathetic other is an important factor in reducing pain levels in specific populations. However, it appears that much depends on the existence of a pre-established bond and strong attachment. One study indicated that the utterance of empathetic statements by trained personnel, who did not previous know the patients, during a painful procedure was not helpful (Lang et al. 2008). Children benefit from the presence of a **supportive other**, as do laboring women. There is extensive research exploring the role of spouses although some spousal behaviors can worsen pain. It appears that the nature of the relationship (attachment) may have a predominant effect on the efficacy of empathetic support in reducing pain (Meredith et al. 2005).

Distraction. Distraction is a well-established approach for the reduction of transient or mild pain (Primack et al. 2012). It is known that playing video games is an effective technique for reducing pain in some populations, especially children (Gold et al. 2006). It is possible that distraction shows a ceiling effect and may not be sufficient for settings where severe pain is anticipated.

Hypnosis. Hypnosis has a long and somewhat rocky association with allopathic medicine. Nonetheless, there is some evidence to support the view that hypnosis is among the interventions that may be useful in mitigating pain. A recent Cochrane database review indicated that self-hypnosis may be beneficial in laboring women (Madden et al. 2016), and a recent study indicated that hypnosis is one of several skills-based psychosocial interventions that may be beneficial for cancer pain [Sheinfeld Gorin]. Importantly, many adults are not hypnotizable whereas children often are. If a patient is open to the idea of hypnosis, a course of therapy may be worthwhile.

Diffuse Noxious inhibitory control. Diffuse Noxious Inhibitory Control (DNIC) is a brain mechanism that suppresses a mild pain when a stronger pain stimulus is encountered. For example, if a person has a scrape on the knee and a broken arm, they may not feel the pain of the knee as long as the arm pain is not controlled. If local measures, e.g. immobilization, icing, nerve blocks, are used to control the arm pain, the patient may become aware of the milder injury to the leg. This has important implications for **multi-trauma** patients as they may not feel all of their injuries and important problems may be overlooked. Many people do not have effective DNIC and a subset of patients experience heightened pain perception in the presence of other pain problems. It is unclear how to utilize DNIC clinically.

Pain Medicine at a Glance, First Edition. Beth B. Hogans.
© 2022 John Wiley & Sons, Ltd. Published 2022 by John Wiley & Sons Ltd.

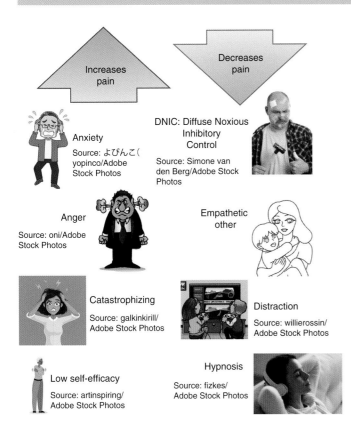

Increases pain

Decreases pain

Anxiety
Source: よぴんこ（yopinco/Adobe Stock Photos

DNIC: Diffuse Noxious Inhibitory Control
Source: Simone van den Berg/Adobe Stock Photos

Anger
Source: oni/Adobe Stock Photos

Empathetic other

Catastrophizing
Source: galkinkirill/Adobe Stock Photos

Distraction
Source: willierossin/Adobe Stock Photos

Low self-efficacy
Source: artinspiring/Adobe Stock Photos

Hypnosis
Source: fizkes/Adobe Stock Photos

References

Burns, J.W., Holly, A., Quartana, P. et al. (2008). Trait anger management style moderates effects of actual ("state") anger regulation on symptom-specific reactivity and recovery among chronic low back pain patients. Psychosomatic Medicine 70: 898–905.

Gold, J.I., Kim, S.H., Kant, A.J. et al. (2006). Effectiveness of virtual reality for pediatric pain distraction during i.v. placement. CyberPsychology and Behaviour 9 (2): 207–212.

Lang, E.V., Berbaum, K.S., Pauker, S.G. et al. (2008). Beneficial effects of hypnosis and adverse effects of empathic attention during percutaneous tumor treatment: when being nice does not suffice. Journal of Vascular and Interventional Radiology 19 (6): 897–905.

Madden K, Middleton P, Cyna AM, Matthewson M, Jones L. Hypnosis for pain management during labour and childbirth. Cochrane Database Syst Rev. 2016 May 19;2016(5):CD009356

Meredith, P.J., Strong, J., and Feeney, J.A. (2005). Evidence of a relationship between adult attachment variables and appraisals of chronic pain. Pain Research and Management 10: 191–200.

Primack, B.A., Carroll, M.V., McNamara, M. et al. (2012). Role of video games in improving health-related outcomes: a systematic review. American Journal of Preventive Medicine 42 (6): 630–638.

Quartana, P.J., Campbell, C.M., and Edwards, R.R. (2009). Pain catastrophizing: a critical review. Expert Review of Neurotherapeutics 9 (5): 745–758.

Rainville, P., Bao, Q.V., and Chrétien, P. (2005). Pain-related emotions modulate experimental pain perception and autonomic responses. Pain 118 (3): 306–318.

Turk, D.C. (2003). Cognitive-behavioral approach to the treatment of chronic pain patients. Regional Anesthesia and Pain Medicine 28 (6): 573–579.

Yarns, B.C., Lumley, M.A., Cassidy, J.T. et al. (2020). Emotional awareness and expression therapy achieves greater pain reduction than cognitive behavioral therapy in older adults with chronic musculoskeletal pain: a preliminary randomized comparison trial. Pain Medicine 21 (11): 2811–2822. 2020 May 25:pnaa145. PMID: 32451528.

8 Approach to the patient with pain: conceptual models of care and related terminology

In treating patients with pain, some conceptual models organize care that is both compassionate and competent. Together, these models provide a robust foundation for approaching the patient in pain.

Balancing treatment and diagnosis: parallel pathway model

The "parallel pathway" model explains the balancing of **diagnostic reasoning** with **compassionate action** (Figure 8.1). Because pain is both a symptom and a cause of suffering, we must attend to patients' need for pain-relief even as diagnosis proceeds. Once we discover pain, we start preliminary pain treatments while simultaneously initiating a diagnostic plan. The parallel pathway model shows how diagnosis and treatment develop in parallel (Murinson et al. 2008). Both are important and time-sensitive. If definitive treatment precedes clear diagnosis, unnecessary harm can occur if we lose the diagnostic information contained in the patient's report of pain. If diagnosis dominates and treatment is delayed while testing takes place, this unnecessarily prolongs suffering. Thus, in the ideal scenario, safe and effective preliminary pain treatments are given, while diagnostic studies are simultaneously undertaken. In the end, "making a diagnosis" will identify disease modifying approaches that more effectively alleviate pain.

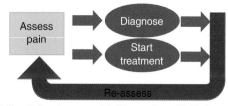

Figure 8.1 Parallel pathway model. Diagnosis and initiation of treatment proceed in parallel so that suffering is relieved as diagnostic efforts are underway.

Understanding pain and choosing rational pharmacotherapy: mechanism based-classification

The mechanism-based classification of pain is a simple yet elegant way to think about pain and pain treatments (Chapter 3). In basic terms, pain arises due to three major pathways: the **nociceptive pathway**, dedicated to sensing injury to the organism; the **inflammatory pathway**, in which sensory endings are sensitized by the action of inflammatory signaling molecules; and the **neuropathic pathway**, which involves an error in nervous system processing of sensory information. Thinking about pain in terms of these mechanisms can 1) elucidate the disease process that is causing the problem, 2) attune us distinctive characteristic qualities associated with each

mechanism which the patient will include in the pain narrative, and 3) guide the design of a treatment plan (Figure 8.2). Most of the pain treatments available are particularly effective for certain mechanisms of pain and less so for other mechanisms. For example, NSAIDs are very useful for treating inflammatory forms of pain; but not effective against neuropathic pain. The management approaches for pain described in this book reflect the conceptual frame that pain is nociceptive, inflammatory, neuropathic, or a combination.

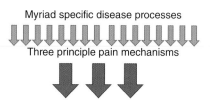

Myriad specific disease processes

Three principle pain mechanisms

Recognizable mechanism-based features

Shared pathophysiology

Shared pharmacological responsiveness

Shared nonpharmacological therapies

Shared Prognostication

Combination for effective treatment of complex conditions

Figure 8.2 Mechanism-based classification of pain overview: rationale for development and how to apply the model.

Patient-centered care vs. disease-centered care

The best pain care balances the needs of the individual patient for pain relief and functional restoration with the providers clinical (disease-specific) knowledge and expectations for healing and recovery

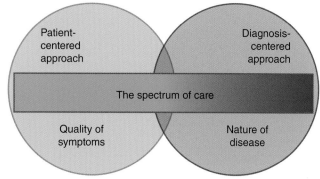

Figure 8.3 Balancing knowledge of disease with patient-centered understanding.

Pain Medicine at a Glance, First Edition. Beth B. Hogans.

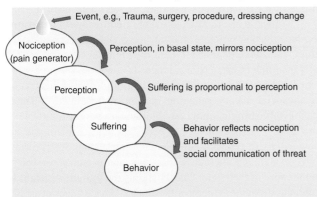

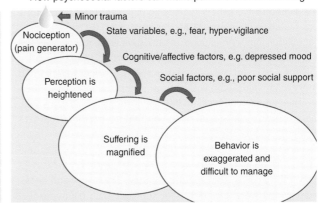

(a) **Biopsychosocial model of pain – normal pain**
Modified to show the pain system normally works

Event, e.g., Trauma, surgery, procedure, dressing change

Nociception (pain generator)

Perception, in basal state, mirrors nociception

Perception

Suffering is proportional to perception

Suffering

Behavior reflects nociception and facilitates social communication of threat

Behavior

(b) **Biopsychosocial model of pain – abberant pain**
How psychosocial factors can make pain more overwhelming

Minor trauma

Nociception (pain generator)

State variables, e.g., fear, hyper-vigilance

Cognitive/affective factors, e.g. depressed mood

Perception is heightened

Social factors, e.g., poor social support

Suffering is magnified

Behavior is exaggerated and difficult to manage

Figure 8.4 (a) Normal functioning demonstrating processes of eudynia; (b) Amplification of pain behavior is a multi-step process (maldynia), this is often associated with the development of chronic pain (Chapter 29). Source: Adapted from Loeser (1982).

(Frankel 2004) (Figure 8.3). This model is related to the parallel pathway model above but highlights that the development of therapeutic approaches needs to incorporate the patient's values and needs, as well as the diagnostic "realities" (Agarwal and Murinson 2012).

Biopsychosocial model

The biopsychosocial model highlights the importance of understanding the patient's psychological and social context which can amplify or diminish pain (Loeser 1982). Like expanding ripples in a pond, dramatic perturbations can arise if frustration builds upon depression upon social isolation to create overwhelming difficulties for the patient who lacks the resources to effectively self-manage pain and pain-related affect (Figure 8.4).

It is in the setting of **persistent** or **chronic** pain that the biopsychosocial model of pain moves to the foreground. The classic scenario is the patient who has been to 20 doctors, takes 12 different medications, relies on pills to start their day and lives from injection to injection. This patient's behavior is dominated by "pain" and their life is ruined in the process.

It is helpful to first examine the case of "normal pain-sensing" or eudynia. **Eudynia** is pain-sensing as a normal function of the nervous system, it is more common than aberrant pain signaling, sometimes termed "**maldynia.**" In eudynia, nociception (primary nociceptive signal transduction) mirrors the degree of injury and is important to ensure survival, Figure 8.2. Each nociception event is mirrored accurately by a perception event. **Perception** is the conscious awareness of pain mediated by the cerebral cortex and leads a person to recognize the potential for injury. The perception of pain is also associated with **suffering**. This affective component of pain, subserved primarily by medial brain structures, such as cingulate cortex, has intrinsic survival value, prompting protective action against further injury. These affective brain centers are tightly linked with learning circuits, causing the organism to remember and avoid potentially injurious settings. The next and

final link in the model is behavior. In normal pain-sensing, behavior mirrors suffering which mirrors perception which mirrors nociception. In eudynia, **pain behavior** serves a useful social purpose of **communicating** a person's pain to those around him or her and is a highly efficient way to solicit help. For example, a child at play falls down and is unharmed, the person watching the child might be alarmed by the fall but immediately recognizes that the child is not crying and must be fine. A scraped knee or broken bone produce various forms of pain behavior that quickly convey the need for attention and aid.

The system breaks down when chronic pain affects a patient with a perturbed psychological state, disrupted mood, and dysfunctional social support network. Minor nociception is amplified by negative cognitions to a more threatening experience of pain, this in the context of depressed mood leads to amplified suffering, and this, in the absence of adequate social supports leads to **aberrant behavior** which disturbs the patient and disrupts those around them. It is impossible to unwind this complex type of pain without coordinated support and collaboration of multiple professionals, all proficient in pain, Chapter 16.

References

Agarwal, A.K. and Murinson, B.B. (2012). New dimensions in patient-physician interaction: values, autonomy, and medical information in the patient-centered clinical encounter. Rambam Maimonides Medical Journal 3 (3): e0017.

Frankel, R.M. (2004). Relationship-centered care and the patient-physician relationship. Journal of General Internal Medicine 19 (11): 1163–1165.

Loeser, J. (1982). Concepts of pain. In: Chronic Low-Back Pain (eds. M. Stanton-Hicks and R. Boas), 145–148. New York: Raven Press.

Murinson, B.B., Agarwal, A.K., and Haythornthwaite, J.A. (2008). Cognitive expertise, emotional development, and reflective capacity: clinical skills for improved pain care. The Journal of Pain 9 (11): 975–983.

9 The pain-focused clinical history: well-developed illness narratives impact pain outcomes

History-taking for the patient with acute pain can focus on eliciting relevant details with empathy and compassion. To build a more durable relationship with patients in persistent pain, it is essential to honor the **pain narrative** by starting with **open questions**, such as: "tell me how your pain began." It is precisely the patient who has told their story many times who will be most impressed by your willingness to listen attentively. In truth, the diagnostic process begins with an illness narrative, embedded there you find the **cardinal features** of the pain. It is imperative to listen with openness and without interrupting, because this is essential to establishing trust (Frankel and Stein 2001). There will never be another opportunity to lay the correct foundation for a robust **therapeutic alliance**. Try to suspend disbelief: perhaps the worst experience for someone with pain is to feel disbelieved. People are exquisitely sensitive to the perception that others are not taking their problems seriously. Don't be the one who leaps to a psychological explanation when genuine pain mechanisms are at work. Small fiber neuropathy is one condition that produces disruptive pain with very few clinical signs. Empathetic demeanor and compassionate concern will elicit gratitude from the patient whose diagnosis remains to be determined (Murinson et al. 2008).

In the pain history, the cardinal features include: **Quality**, **Region**, **Severity**, and **Timing**. It is also helpful to elicit: what is "Usually associated with" the pain, what steps have made the pain "Very much better," and what has made the pain "Worse," Table 9.1. Pain severity can be rapidly assessed with a standard scale (Figure 9.1). It is sometimes necessary to establish the cardinal features of more than one "pain." For example, patients with headaches often experience multiple headache types; each should be characterized and may require different therapy.

In the acute setting, the pain history may be quite brief. In this context, the **biomedical model** is relevant: what are the **proximate** causes of a pain problem, what are the pertinent medical conditions. Clinically, we think in terms of "finding a **pain generator**," i.e., locating the primary afferent nerve endings activated by an injury. The quick pain history and the biomedical model are typically insufficient when pain is longer lasting.

In the chronic pain setting, the insightful provider finds that **biopsychosocial** history gathering is often more effective. Time is spent **establishing rapport** and building a relationship (Cole and Bird 2013). The patient with a persistent pain problem will have more extensive **relevant experience**: prior testing, interventional, conventional, and alternative therapies, and personal perspectives on the cause of their pain. Understanding the **patient's insight** into their pain strengthens therapeutic alliance (McCormack et al. 2013) (Figure 9.2). Recognizing what the patient values and genuinely enjoys in life becomes essential when implementing a **chronic disease model** to change behavior, as is necessary in managing persistent pain-associated conditions. Knowing that patient wants to return to specific sports, hobbies, or work-related activities will make discussions of "engagement in physical therapy" or "maintaining a moderate exercise program" more successful, couched in terms of returning to valued activities. This is referred to as motivational interviewing, discussed later (Miller and Rollnick 2002).

For those with **cognitive impairments** and **dementia**, it is important to utilize situationally appropriate observations. Pain behaviors in older adults can include irritability, social isolation, grimacing, groaning, sweating, tachypnea, tachycardia, guarding, and limping. For more detail, see Chapter 51.

For **children**, it is important to conduct an **age-appropriate pain assessment**. Children over the age of 7 should be assessed for capacity to utilize the numerical rating scale. From 4 to 7 the FACES scale is more appropriate. Infants and pre-verbal children

Table 9.1 Pain alphabet.

Pain
Quality
Region
Severity
Timing
Usually associated with
Very much better with
Worse with

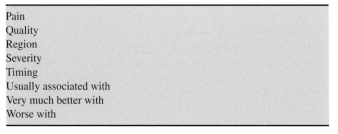

Figure 9.1 The numerical rating scale.

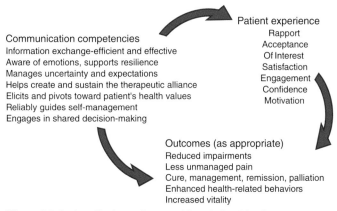

Figure 9.2 In the effective patient-provider relationship, there are many forms of communication, patient experiences, and potential outcomes that impact pain care.

Pain Medicine at a Glance, First Edition. Beth B. Hogans.

require behavioral pain scales such as the FLACC and the NIPS. Please see Chapter 50 for more details.

Emotional impact

Some patients will become irritable when socioemotional barriers are explored. Others will express sincere appreciation that you want to understand their experiences more fully. By empathetically entering into the patient's experience you can lighten their burden while fostering genuine connection that will be a strong foundation for future progress (Rogers 1967). More in Chapter 10.

Sleep

The quality and quantity of sleep has a direct and profound influence on pain persistence and severity. It is critical to ask about sleep at the initial visit and to check back about sleep quality and quantity at subsequent visits, see Chapter 25 for details.

Function

Pain has a profound effect on multiple domains of function as noted in Chapter 1, Figure 1.3. Functional assessment in patients with pain, usually focuses on specific domains, noted here in Table 9.2.

Table 9.2 Pain functional interference.

Does pain interfere with your:
"Work at home"?
"Work at work"?
Care for self?
Relationships with family?
Friendships?
Social or civic activities?
Enjoyment of life?
Sleep?
Mood?

Biopsychosocial model

The degree to which the patient will recognize aspects of the biopsychosocial model is expediently explored with an educational handout about the model. The patient, once introduced to the concepts, see Chapter 8, is presented with a check list, such as that in Table 9.3, providing the opportunity to endorse multiple complicating factors.

Openness to treatments – foundations of MI

A useful way to assess openness to treatments is, besides asking the patient what treatments they are interested in, is to use a check sheet as part of the check-in or counseling process. See Chapter 16 and Appendix 5.

Table 9.3 Biopsychosocial model: with examples for each Bio – Psycho – Social model: the details.

Biological	Psychological	Social
Disc/vertebral degeneration	Depression	Smoking
Facet joint arthritis	Anxiety	Poor ergonomics
Ingrowth of pain-type nerve endings	PTSD	Lack of exercise
Ligamentous stretch or hypertrophy	Post-TBI	Stress
Muscle strain	Other mental illness	Physical demands
Radiculopathy	Dysphoria	Poor sleep
Altered central pain processing	Somatic focus	De-conditioning
	Low self-efficacy	Lack of social support
	Substance abuse	Expectations
	Personality d/o	

Social history and work–life

The role of professional work–life in the social history has fallen from vogue but serves a central purpose in understanding the patient's everyday jargon and **cognitive frame**.

A check-in form (or tablet protocol) that efficiently assesses pain can allow a provider to track changes over time, screen for opioid abuse risk, and provide valuable diagnostic information, in addition to conveying information about other prescription medicines, dietary supplements, exercise patterns, social habits, and comorbid conditions.

References

Cole, S.A. and Bird, J. (2013). The Medical Interview: The Three Function Approach with Student Consult Online Access, 3e. Philadelphia, PA: Saunders.

Frankel, R.M. and Stein, T. (2001). Getting the most out of the clinical encounter: the four habits. The Journal of Medical Practice Management 16 (4): 184–191.

McCormack, L., Treiman, K., Olmsted, M. et al. (2013). Advancing Measurement of Patient-Centered Communication in Cancer Care. Effective Health Care Program Research Report No. 39. (Prepared by RTI DEcIDE Center under Contract No. 290- 2005-0036-I.) AHRQ Publication No. 12(13)-EHC057-EF. Rockville, MD: Agency for Healthcare Research and Quality.

Miller, W.R. and Rollnick, S. (2002). Motivational Interviewing: Preparing People for Change, 2e. New York: Guilford Press.

Murinson, B.B., Agarwal, A.K., and Haythornthwaite, J.A. (2008). Cognitive expertise, emotional development, and reflective capacity: clinical skills for improved pain care. The Journal of Pain 9 (11): 975–983.

Rogers, C. (1967). The interpersonal relationship in the facilitation of learning. In: Humanizing Education (ed. R. Leeper), 1–18. Alexandria, VA: Association for Supervision and Curriculum Development.

In those with communication barriers, pain assessment requires adaptations depending on the nature of the barrier.

Speech barriers

Speech barriers can include dysarthria, aphasia, and developmental disturbances of speech. **Dysarthria** is a motor difficulty in speech production that makes it difficult to understand what a person is saying but without cognitive defects consider writing, picture boards, or alternative words. Dysarthria may arise from damage to the **right frontal region** which can also result in **personality changes** making people more critical and less flexible. These personality changes can frustrate family members and may lead to behavioral challenges. Conversely, **expressive aphasia** reflects dysfunction of the left frontal lobe, it limits a patient's ability to verbalize what they wish to communicate, they will know what they want to say and can understand instructions well, these patients can participate effectively in physical therapy. **Receptive aphasia**, in which patients cannot understand what is being said, is more challenging as patients cannot always understand instructions and depending on the baseline personality may have variable inclinations to mimic gestures by cueing. There are more complex aphasias as well. Unfortunately, patients with aphasia often cannot communicate through written mediums. In this case, pain assessment may be limited to behavioral assessments. It is feasible in this context to utilize gentle provocative testing to elicit relevant pain features. For example, rebound tenderness in the abdomen will still produce the clinically relevant response. A systematic effort to uncover painful areas, painful movements, or pain on palpation may be the best available information. Sometimes pantomiming, drawing pictures or bringing **pictures** up on the computer screen can elicit the bright smile of understanding from a patient who is otherwise withdrawn and absorbed in morose frustration.

Hearing barriers

These may be surmountable using communication tools: written questionnaires, computer assistance, or a **signing interpreter**. If a patient has not been formally educated, as can happen in low resource countries, a family member may be essential for communicating in the "home language." Be aware that patients may nod to indicate receptiveness not necessarily understanding or assent. It is important to check for understanding affirmatively despite communication barriers.

Language barriers

The use of professional translation is preferred for obtaining a multidimensional pain history. Family members should generally not provide translation services as there is a complex interaction between culture and pain communication.

Socioemotional barriers

Some patients have psychological or socioemotional barriers to communicating about pain. Clinically-diagnosed malingering and factitious disorder are rare; addiction can be associated with manipulation of clinical findings but this is complex (Chapter 46). Occasional patients are reluctant to return to work, attempt to assuage difficulties with medication, or simply wish to have more time off. More commonly, patients reporting persistent pain have not experienced sufficient therapeutic relief or functional improvement to resume normal activity. It is important to establish a differential diagnosis and support rehabilitation in a structured manner. Noncompliance with an appropriate therapy plan should be addressed in an **open** and **accountable** manner as psychological or psychiatric disturbance often underlies failure to engage appropriately in treatment and should be addressed appropriately for optimal outcomes. Documentation is key.

Managing affect and negotiating boundaries with pain patients

Patients with pain are highly motivated to seek pain relief and those with chronic pain often have some degree of anger or frustration with the medical system for real or perceived failings. One common feature that unites almost every patient with pain is an eagerness for someone to listen to their illness narrative and vigorously pursue solutions to their problem. Some patients, especially those who have been very frustrated by previous medical experiences, may be impatient with students and younger physicians (Murinson et al. 2008) (Figure 10.1). Too often, patients with chronic pain have been told that nothing can be done. Others have become dependent on pain medicines or recurrent procedures and have fallen into a role of **passivity** and **conditioned behavior**. Some patients have experienced healthcare harms. All these may be suspicious until a healthy therapeutic alliance is built.

Remember that **safety of patient and provider** is the primary concern in any clinical setting. If a patient is overly personal, aggressive, or threatening, seek help immediately (Figure 10.2). Curse words or a harsh tone of voice may be early signs of an evolving hostile state, it is important to maintain an atmosphere of **mutual respect** and insist that the **boundaries** of a professional relationship are respected. Patients who are seeking opioids from a position of dependency will sometimes be overly agreeable or flattering, Exercise caution with the patient who seems too nice, showering you or your staff with compliments, gifts, or favors. Receipt of gifts and acceptance of personal favors is not acceptable as this undermines the provider's ethical stance. Remember that in many patients, some **resistance** to a new idea may signal the **change process** is starting, indicating that the patient is engaging and seriously considering behavior change. Some patients have difficulty expressing emotions, these patients may

Pain Medicine at a Glance, First Edition. Beth B. Hogans.
© 2022 John Wiley & Sons Ltd. Published 2022 by John Wiley & Sons Ltd.

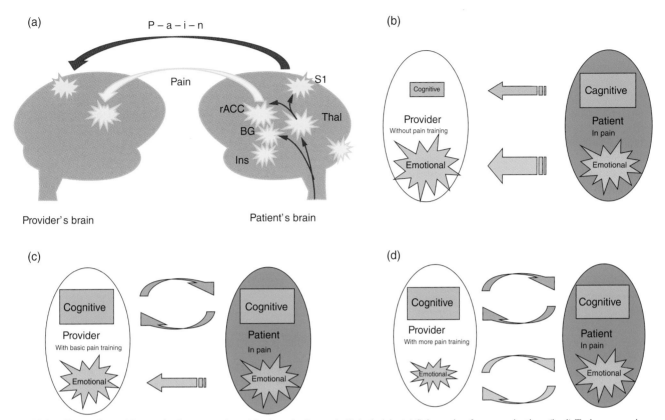

Figure 10.1 Affect and cognition are both communicated in the pain-focused clinical visit. (a) Schematic of communication. (b–d) Trainees acquire skillfulness in managing cognitive information and enhancing the affective dimensions of the interaction. This develops from unidirectional (b) to effective cognitive communication, reducing affective overloading (c) to effective, bidirectional communication that is supportive of patient and rewarding for provider. Source: Adapted from Murinson (2015) and Murinson et al. (2008).

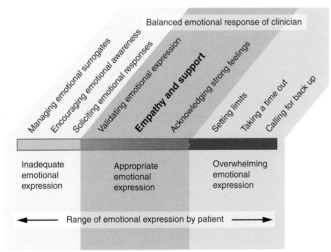

Figure 10.2 Recognizing and modulating the emotional range of a pain-focused clinical visit.

need support from you to open to their feelings, a reflective statement such as "It seems like this might be really hard for you" can give the patient permission to share and can help a clinician identify specific ways to help (Roter et al. 2006). "Cognitive impairment is addressed in Chapter 51, pediatric pain assessment

in Chapter 50, and pain assessment in the context of medication or drug dependence in Chapter 46."

In summary, communication barriers to pain assessment take many forms. Some pertain to the mechanics of communication while others primarily impact the affective dimensions. Openness, skill, adaptability, and compassion are necessary in building a therapeutic alliance to overcome pain.

References

Murinson, B. (2015). Expertise, skillfulness and professional comportment: preparing clinical trainees for effectiveness in pain care. Invited lecture at Pain Research, Education and Policy Program, Tufts School of Medicine, Boston, Massachusetts. https://www.youtube.com/watch?v=L_pY7cTDygs (accessed 20 December 2017).

Murinson, B.B., Agarwal, A.K., and Haythornthwaite, J.A. (2008). Cognitive expertise, emotional development, and reflective capacity: clinical skills for improved pain care. The Journal of Pain 9 (11): 975–983.

Roter, D.L., Frankel, R.M., Hall, J.A., and Sluyter, D. (2006). The expression of emotion through nonverbal behavior in medical visits. Mechanisms and outcomes. Journal of General Internal Medicine 21 (Suppl 1): S28–S34. Review.

11 Examination skills I: interaction, observation, and affect

The desire to benefit mankind deeply motivates most who enter clinical work. Examining patients with pain brings skills, interest, and empathy into play at once. There is an essential difference between the expedient clinician who forcefully compresses a painful area, compared with the kindly one who first presses on a non-tender spot, accommodating the patient to the feeling of normal pressure, and attentively checks for the patient's response while advancing towards the area of expected pain. Some have been acculturated to think it's not cool to attend to pain, but you may already know that listening to and looking for pain give valuable clues to diagnosis. This chapter is about looking for pain and its concomitants.

Observation

Patients have certain behaviors in response to pain that vary as pain changes from hyperacute to acute to chronic (Table 11.1). In the *hyperacute phase*, i.e., at the time of injury, people may not feel the pain they will inevitably later. Those injuries that we witness at sporting events, for example, may not initially manifest all they pain that ultimately pertains to the injury. Some of this comes from descending inhibition mechanisms and activation of the HPA axis.

In the *acute phase*, people have fairly predictable behaviors in response to pain: these behaviors are useful to the examiner. If you watch when a painful part is pressed or moved, you will see a range of pain behaviors including guarding, wincing, and vocalization. **Guarding** is a motor adaptation to pain: body posture, head position, movement of the limbs changes in response to acute pain. If a limb is painful, the patient may hold the limb toward the body, even curl the body around the limb defensively. Pain in the head may be accompanied by hunching posture, head holding, and tension in the shoulders. Picture what this person would look like if they were happy and carefree, then describe the observable differences.

Table 11.1 Pain behaviors by temporal phase.

Hyperacute behaviors	Early phase behaviors	Late phase behaviors
"Smile of pain"	Wincing	Sometimes no expression
Shock	Guarding	Reliance of passive strategies
Stunned silence	Vocalization	Social isolation

Source: TheVisualsYouNeed/Adobe Stock Photos

Source: blvdone/Adobe Stock Photos

Guarding is very useful to the clinician because changes in body mechanics are often present even with mild pain and guarding is often subconscious. Tensing, clenching, or pulling away are other spontaneous motor pain responses. Next time you see a jogger, take a few minutes to appreciate whether there are gait perturbations potentially reflecting misuse or injuries.

Wincing can be a spontaneous response and should be noted. Facial cues provoked by pain can also be a learned social behavior and may be useful to prompt the clinician to empathetically ask: "does that hurt?" and ask permission to proceed. Wincing may be overwrought in someone trying to gain sympathy but this is relatively rare and comes along with other signs of manipulation.

Vocalization is typically reserved for moderate to severe pain. The seasoned obstetrician will recognize changes in a woman's voice when she enters the final phases of labor. Vocalizations range from cheek puffing, a sharp intake of air, to plosives such as "ay," "oy," and "ow," to outright cries and screams. Vocalizations are culturally dependent and should be responded to calmly. Vocalizations are often spontaneous and may represent a genuine perception of pain by the patient.

Chronic pain can be surprisingly devoid of pain behavior

For years researchers believed that "there is no pain behavior." This is simply not true in the acute phase, where clear and consistent acute pain behaviors reflect deeply established motor patterns in the brain (Jasmin et al. 1997). Chronic pain manifests an entirely different set of behaviors, some learned and some intrinsic. People make remarkable adaptations to living with chronic pain but often, careful observation of behavior will lend essential clues to understanding the medical circumstances.

Affect

Emotion and affect are important dimensions that profoundly impact outcomes. **Affect** is the "conscious subjective aspect of an emotion considered apart from bodily changes" (Mirriam-Webster 1828). It is palpable to the astute observer. The first step is to **name the emotion** that you believe present (Table 11.2). Next is to **gauge appropriateness**, silently and internally, of the perceived emotional response, this is part of emotional intelligence (Murinson et al. 2008) (Figure 11.1). Then, you will respond, potentially offering a **supportive response**: a spoken empathetic phrase or an appropriate wordless vocalization, in either case accompanied by non-defensive **body language**. Even patients that are expressing hostility will respond better to appropriately supportive responses although boundary setting may be necessary if being supportive is not sufficient. If a patient is exhibiting hostile range of affect, you will need to think about **safety** concerns and next steps. If sorrow, acceptance, frustration, or positive emotions are expressed, more reflective responses are appropriate. If a patient's affect is

Pain Medicine at a Glance, First Edition. Beth B. Hogans.
© 2022 John Wiley & Sons Ltd. Published 2022 by John Wiley & Sons Ltd.

Table 11.2 Management of affect NURSE acronym.

Name the feeling – It sounds like you're feeling disappointed
Understand – I can understand how these feelings come up
Respect – You have been really brave through all this
Support – We will figure out together (build an alliance)
Explore – What is it that bothers you the most?

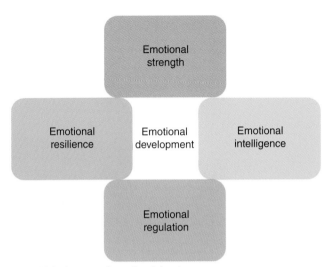

Figure 11.1 Aspects of emotional development.

excessively flat or muted, this may also be cause for concern. Humor can be used carefully to shape the emotional tone of an encounter but should be avoided when a patient is irritable, hostile or angry. If a patient is generally genial in their demeanor, humor can useful to smooth over any minor glitches. Mild self-deprecating humor is well tolerated. Humor that singles out others for ridicule should be strictly avoided. The best way to establish a strong, **trusting rapport** with a patient is to sit down with them as you listen to their illness (pain) narrative (Back et al. 2005). Make sure to have open body language: lean forward slightly, do not cross arms or legs, and maintain a neutral, slightly pleasant facial expression. Generally, good eye contact is positive unless there are precluding cultural factors. A patient that feels listened to and understood will be satisfied and this emotional connection will lead to improved health outcomes (Stein et al. 2005).

References

Back, A.L., Arnold, R.M., Baile, W.F. et al. (2005). Approaching difficult communication tasks in oncology. CA: a Cancer Journal for Clinicians 55 (3): 164–177.

Jasmin, L., Burkey, A.R., Card, J.P., and Basbaum, A.I. (1997). Transneuronal labeling of a nociceptive pathway, the spino-(trigemino-)parabrachio-amygdaloid, in the rat. The Journal of Neuroscience 17 (10): 3751–3765.

Mirriam-Webster (1828). Mirriam-Webster dictionary. https://www.merriam-webster.com/dictionary/affect (accessed 1 October 2017).

Murinson, B.B., Agarwal, A.K., and Haythornthwaite, J.A. (2008). Cognitive expertise, emotional development, and reflective capacity: clinical skills for improved pain care. The Journal of Pain 9 (11): 975–983.

Stein, T., Frankel, R.M., and Krupat, E. (2005). Enhancing clinician communication skills in a large healthcare organization: a longitudinal case study. Patient Education and Counseling 58 (1): 4–12.

Examination is a vital moment in the patient-provider relationship. The young clinician faces many challenges as they establish skillfulness: conducting the motor aspects of examination, learning to recognize and retain important clinical findings, collecting additional items from the pain-focused history, and maintaining a comfortable relaxed rapport with the patient. In addition, gentle and considerate conduct is often more effortful than being quick and forceful. Nonetheless, patients respect and value caring and kindness coupled with knowledge and skill. This inspiration and respect will translate into patient satisfaction and engagement in treatment.

Inspection

Inspection is the astute clinician's most valuable tool. Forgo this step out of embarrassment or expediency at peril. Looking at a painful part will often clinch a diagnosis or exclude several relevant ones. For example: pain radiating down the leg may be suspected radiculopathy, most typically not associated with any visible changes in the acute phase (although the observational changes to gait may be obvious). If you lift the sheet and see a swollen, red leg, the differential diagnosis shifts radically toward vascular and infectious causes. With inspection you are looking for asymmetry, swelling, coloration, and integrity of skin, hair, and nails.

Palpation

Palpation should proceed with care. Although seemingly quick to press firmly on the diagnostic point of greatest interest, this will not promote a meaningful patient-provider relationship. It is preferable to **palpate non-painful parts first** so that the patient can accommodate to the feeling of non-painful pressure and establish trust that the provider is careful in touching them. This is a way to show respect for a patient's dignity as a person. Palpation should be with the pads of the fingers and proceed toward the area of maximal anticipated pain. Masses and edema are noted, and their extent, size, quality, and location described or diagramed (LeBlond and Brown 2014) (Figure 12.1). Thermal qualities of the relevant areas should be assessed. It is critical to recall that the pads of the fingers and the palms of the hands do not have the same density of **heat receptors** as are present on the **back of the hand**. Therefore, when determining the thermal features, e.g. heat or cold in an area,

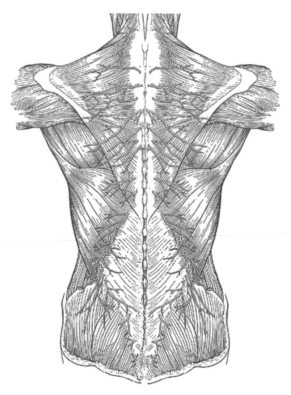

Figure 12.1 Anatomical posterior view of the torso. Source: Adapted from Gray's anatomy (1918, public source), adapted by BBH.

it is necessary to turn the hand over and apply the dorsum (back) of the middle and proximal phalanges to the patient's skin. Then your thermal receptors will be able to perceive the temperature of the patient's skin much more effectively.

Range of motion

Range of motion (ROM) is assessed both in terms of passive and active range. Some general ROM values are noted in Table 12.1. **Passive ROM** is tested when the examiner moves the part for the patient. **Active ROM** is tested when the patient does the moving. Depending on the condition, either or both may be important. ROM is often limited by pain and this should be noted.

Table 12.1 Range of motion of commonly tested parts.

Neck flexion	Neck extension	Neck side flexion	Neck rotation	Arm abduction	Elbow flexion	Back flexion at waist	Back extension	Hip flexion	Knee flexion
50	80	45	85	180	145	55	15	125	140

Pain Medicine at a Glance, First Edition. Beth B. Hogans.
© 2022 John Wiley & Sons Ltd. Published 2022 by John Wiley & Sons Ltd.

Motor testing

Motor testing is accomplished in order to shape the **differential diagnosis** and inform an assessment of the patient's **impairment**. Proper technique is absolutely essential. In order to assess a muscle, the clinician must have an understanding of the muscular anatomy and function so that the muscle can be isolated and tested for strength. A table of commonly tested muscles is provided here (Table 12.2). For more details, the reader may consult a specialty reference (O'Brien 2010).

Table 12.2 Selected muscle name and innervation levels.

Rhomboid	Deltoid	Biceps	Triceps	Wrist extensors	APB	ADV
C5	C5-6	C5-6	C6-7-8	C6-7-8	C8/T1	C8/T1
Iliopsoas	**Adductors**	**Quadriceps**	**Hamstrings**	**Tib. Ant.**	**Gastroc.**	**Add. Hall.**
L1-2-3-4	L2-3-4-5	L2-3-4-5	L4-5/S1-2	L4-5/S1	L5/S1-2	S1-2

Sensory testing

Sensory testing is necessary depending on the pain-associated conditions that are under consideration. For nerve conditions such as radiculopathy, neuropathy, and spinal cord injury, sensory testing is essential. Sensory testing may include light touch but more often for pain conditions, the perception of a sharp stimulus is most informative. The technique of **testing sharp sensation** is important. The use of "safety pins" is strongly discouraged. Safety pins may draw blood unnecessarily. Use of a sharply broken wooden applicator stick or use of precision-made sharp testing pins (Neurotip) is acceptable, see Chapter 45. There is some controversy about testing methods but patients may have increased sensation to sharp stimuli (hyperalgesia) or decreased sensation. **Hyperalgesia** is often observed in neuropathic and inflammatory conditions. Pressure on the sharp object should be "just right," too much may pierce the skin, too little will not be sufficient to provoke a sharp sensation. Tapping with the sharp object may be used to elicit **aberrant temporal summation**, a useful sign of small fiber peripheral neuropathy.

Special senses testing is necessary depending on the pain-associated condition under consideration. For headache especially it is necessary to evaluate visual function with care as brain tumors may manifest with insidious headache and a subtle visual field deficit unnoticed by the patient. When testing visual fields, it is better for the patient count fingers rather than detect finger wiggling. This is because motion is detected at the level of the brainstem whereas perceptual vision mediating finger counting is a cortical task: the intended target of this test. Hearing may be important for head pain, especially with other cranial neuropathies. Taste testing may be important for conditions such as burning mouth syndrome.

Reflex testing

Reflex testing is necessary depending on the pain-associated conditions that are under consideration. For nerve conditions such as radiculopathy, neuropathy, and spinal cord injury, reflex testing is non-negotiable (Figure 12.2). Reflexes are often used to *exclude* nerve involvement; however this is inaccurate as tested reflexes survey a very limited number of nerve root levels (Table 12.3).

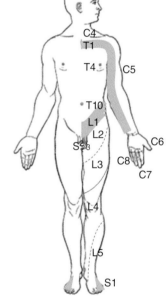

Figure 12.2 Dermatomes on male figure. Developed by the author (BBH) from public domain drawing (Grays 1918), with dermatomes from Duus, Netter, and AccessAnesthesiology, composite information.

Table 12.3 Reflex testing.

Reflex	Level
Biceps	C5-6
Brachioradialis	C5-6
Triceps	C7-8
Patella	L3-4
Ankle	S1-2

Provocative testing

Provocative testing varies depending on the syndrome under consideration. Provocative tests are popular because they can dramatically advance diagnostic thinking and have been studied from an evidenced based perspective, see Chapters 31–45.

References

Gray, H. (1918). Anatomy of the Human Body. Philadelphia: Lea & Febiger; Bartleby.com, 2000. www.bartleby.com/107/.

LeBlond, R. and Brown, D. (2014). DeGowin's Diagnostic Examination, 10e (Lange)Sep 5. New York: McGraw-Hill.

O'Brien, M. (2010). Aids to the Examination of the Peripheral Nervous System, 5e. Philadelphia, PA: Saunders.

For decades pain medicine was propelled forward by the belief that those provided with sufficient knowledge would become capable practitioners. Due to the slow adoption of pain in general clinical education, most practitioners have never attained adequate pain knowledge. An additional difficulty comes in ensuring that patients receive care that is **knowledgeable** and **skillful** and **compassionate**. The capacity of a curriculum to transmit compassionate care practices is a challenge that may be met in the twenty-first century with new standards in **assessment**, **practice**, and **competency**. Requiring trainees to pass validated observed examinations, called Objective Standardized Clinical Exams, or OSCEs (oss-keys) for short is currently popular. OSCEs hold the promise of observing behaviors that are associated with efficient diagnosis: attention to patients' values and effective shared decision-making talk. It is difficult to rate a provider on empathy and compassion, but efforts are made using **observation checklists**. Despite these limitations, experienced pain practitioners rate "compassionate care practices" as the most important aspect of pain medicine to be transmitted to trainees (Murinson et al. 2013). In this chapter, we explore resources for expanding knowledge, skills, and compassionate practices pertaining to pain care.

The knowledge base of clinical medicine has expanded and solidified dramatically in the years since the birth of modern pain medicine in the 1970s. **John Bonica**, an American anesthesiologist and semi-pro wrestler originally published "The Management of Pain" in 1953, now available as a highly-rated 5th edition (Ballantyne et al. 2018). He went on to found the **International Association for the Study of Pain (IASP)** in 1972 at age 55. Both his book, now in a fourth edition and his organization, now over 7000 members representing 133 countries a full spectrum of professions, continue to be important sources of cutting edge knowledge about pain. IASP publishes a seminal research journal "Pain" as well as open source publications dedicated to disseminating evidence based clinical information about pain. Biannual meetings are held by IASP. In the United States, the US Association for the Study of Pain (USASP) is the official IASP chapter. The **American Academy of Pain Medicine** hosts an annual educational conference targeting pain-interested clinicians, with tracks for pain interventionalists, general practitioners (**MDs, PAs, CRNPs**), and to military (**VA/DoD**) medicine. There are national specialty (anesthesia), regional and proprietary conferences, and online certificate programs. In 1988, the IASP published a curriculum for entry level pain education (Pilowsky 1988). Later, time-contingent curricular recommendations were promulgated by the **European Federation of IASP Chapters, EFIC**, specifying 40 hours of instruction, highly ambitious for most health professions schools (EFIC 2004). By the early 2000s, studies in Canada, the U.S. and elsewhere indicated that most medical schools were far below this target (Mezei and Murinson 2011; Watt-Watson et al. 2009). Recommendations

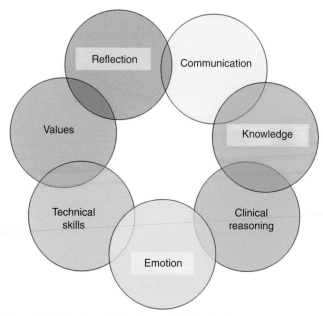

Figure 13.1 Epstein and Hundert model of professional competence is based on multiple spheres of proficiency. Management of emotion, knowledge, and reflection are especially important in the pain-focused clinical encounter.

from the AAPM followed in 2012 (Murinson et al. 2013). IASP has now revised its educational guidance into interprofessional and uni-professional curricular curricula, and competencies have been proposed (Fishman et al. 2013).

The **technical skills** required for pain clinical care vary depending on a provider's focus. Some PCPs want to perform basic procedures. There is a strong trend towards visualization in all areas of procedural management. Ultrasound has become increasing popular for basic injections and fluoroscopy is now standard-of-care for many if not most of the injections given by procedural pain medicine specialists. Procedural skills require appropriate training and continuous practice.

Besides interventional skills, there are numerous cognitive and affective skills in pain medicine. **Epstein and Hundert** defined **clinical competence** as consisting of seven domains in their landmark article on clinical competence (Epstein and Hundert 2002, Fig. 13.1). A general practitioner will need skill in assessing pain, this can include having a pain-focused interface available to the patient at check in, saving valuable time in the visit to focus on building rapport, eliciting the narrative, physical examination, and shared decision making: tasks requiring clinical skillfulness. Incorporating relevant forms of non-pharmacological treatment, and formulating and communicating a safe and effective pharmacological treatment plan also requires skillfulness. These are tasks that improve with effort and practice but exposure to excellent role models and training opportunities are essential.

Pain Medicine at a Glance, First Edition. Beth B. Hogans.
© 2022 John Wiley & Sons Ltd. Published 2022 by John Wiley & Sons Ltd.

Figure 13.2 Dimensions of emotional competence: applied to pain care. Source: Based on Murinson et al. 2010.

Emotional strength	
Empathy	Vicarious experience of the thoughts, feelings or actions of another
Compassion	Awareness of the suffering of another coupled with the desire to relieve that suffering
Capacity	Ability to experience loss and to celebrate success

Emotional regulation	
Prioritization	Placing the needs of others over self when appropriate
Conscientiousness	A sense duty and willingness to work diligently
Delay of gratification	Ability to postpone rewards

Emotional intelligence	
Perception	Awareness of emotions in self and others
Anticipation	Knows of and can pre-sage "normal" emotional reactions
Recognition	Distinguishes aberrant emotional reactions

Emotional resilience	
Attentive to self-care	Maintenance of emotional reserves
Flexible	Tolerance of uncertainty or ambiguity
Self-healing	Ability to restore balance and attain positive perspectives
Calm and capable	Capacity to de-escalate emotionally charged situations

Compassionate practices in pain clinical care are often given the short shrift in education despite central importance to the patient's experience. It is hard to imagine what compels a provider to say: "You have the spine of a ninety-year-old". Imagine the patient hearing this: a pervasive sense of hopelessness, embarrassment, and fear that nothing can be done. It is critically important to give patients hope that some aspect of their condition is treatable. It may be obvious to a patient that they cannot return to perfect functioning, but "harsh truths" rarely produce desirable changes, they only produce feelings of disappointment with the provider who leveled such a negative appraisal. Consideration for other is sometimes conveyed in the Golden Rule as "Do unto others as you would have done unto you." Usefully, the rule has been alternatively stated as "Do not do unto another that which is hateful to you." This may be an especially useful and pragmatic reformulation: although we cannot always provide the ideal clinical experience, we can certainly avoid saying or doing things that diminish another person's sense of their own human value. In the ideal world, we would contextualize compassion training in a broader context of socioemotional development. One formulation of this derives from emotional intelligence research and is presented in Figure 13.2. Our health professions education goal is to **promote self-efficacy and self-management in a respectful and appreciative manner**. The comprehensive pain care model (Chapter 16) developed in parallel with the comprehensive clinical competence model described here. We envision that a competent and (socioemotionally) actualized health professional will be highly effective in negotiating and supporting pain self-management for their patients. What is more compassionate than cheering on a patient's efforts and success in improving their own health? This is a formula for better patient outcomes, and lower rates of **provider burnout** – a double bonus.

References

Ballantyne, J.C., Fishman, S.M., and Rathmell, J.P. (2018). Bonica's Management of Pain, 5e. Philadelphia, PA: Wolters Kluwer.

Epstein, R.M. and Hundert, E.M. (2002). Defining and assessing professional competence. JAMA 287: 226–235.

European Federation of IASP Chapters (2004). Draft proposal for a core curriculum for undergraduate medical education. http://www.efic.org/edu-draft-proposal. php (accessed 23 August 2010).

Fishman, S.M., Young, H.M., Lucas Arwood, E. et al. (2013). Core competencies for pain management: results of an interprofessional consensus summit. Pain Medicine 14 (7): 971–981.

Mezei, L. and Murinson, B.B.; Johns Hopkins Pain Curriculum Development Team (2011). Pain education in North American medical schools. Journal of Pain 12 (12): 1199–1208.

Murinson, B.B., Sutton, T.J., and Buenaver, L.F. (2010). Emotional development in the context of pain and the humanities. IASP 13th World Congress, Montreal, Quebec Canada.

Murinson, B.B., Gordin, V., Driver, L. et al. (2013). Recommendations for a new curriculum in pain medicine for medical students: towards a career distinguished by competence and compassion. Pain Medicine 14 (3): 345–350.

Pilowsky, I. (1988). An outline curriculum on pain for medical schools. Pain 33: 1–2.

Watt-Watson, J., McGillion, M., Hunter, J. et al. (2009). A survey of prelicensure pain curricula in health science faculties in Canadian universities. Pain Research and Management 14 (6): 439–444.

14 Motivational interviewing and shared decision-making: psychological skills in primary care for pain

Traditional models of clinical care, unchanged since Hippocrates, envision a seasoned clinician transmitting decisions, by edict or persuasion, to a patient who must at all costs comply with recommendations. These have been supplanted by more adaptable models of patient-clinician interaction. As described by Emmanuel and Emmanuel, the traditional model involved low patient autonomy but with the protean social changes arising the post-World War era, some patients expressed a strong preference for high levels of autonomy (Emanuel and Emanuel 1992). Today the landscape of **patient-provider interactions** is considerably more complex, and providers must quickly assess a patient's desire for autonomy and proceed accordingly whilst maintaining a willingness to shift to higher or lower autonomy modes as new information accrues or awareness of the patient's preferences changes. As noted by Agarwal and Murinson, patients also vary in terms of their desire to engage in healthcare-related decisions on the basis of **independent knowledge acquisition**, and the extent to which they hold **strong health-related values**, i.e. some patients will refuse transfusion on religious grounds (Agarwal and Murinson 2012). That said, the general trend is towards a presumption of **high autonomy** on the part of patients with providers increasingly filling a role of **education** and **decision-support**. There are circumstances such as trauma-care in which the default position is one of low autonomy as life-saving efforts supersede other considerations.

Often providers are in the position of knowing that a particular health-related choice is clearly in the patient's best interest clinically, e.g. smoking cessation, weight loss, moderate exercise, physical therapy, and yet, the patient does not follow through on recommendations that are made. These challenges have been addressed for many different conditions as part of a **chronic disease model paradigm**, Table 14.1. The answers depend on who you ask: economists propose providing financial incentives, public health graduates encourage systemic solutions such as water filtration; and employers offer discounts for gym memberships and body mass index goals. Often, clinicians feel frustrated when patients return 5 pounds heavier and smelling of cigarette smoke. There are *evidence based approaches for promoting behavior change*, the most relevant and widespread are **motivational interviewing** and the **Stages of Change model** (Prochaska et al. 1992; Miller and Rollnick 2002).

A first step in this process is exploring the **patient's values**. It is important to know about the patient's social support system: work, family, friends, and social activities. It may also be helpful to know the patient's career interests, this facilitates understanding their cognitive frame. When it is necessary to provide an explanation for a problem that the patient is having, it's helpful to have access to their day-to-day jargon. An electrician, will readily grasp neuropathic pain described as a "short in the system" whereas for a bus driver, it might be helpful to describe a busy street where people are

Table 14.1 Behavior change in healthcare: comparison of models.

Stage in stages of change model	Patient state	Other models
Pre-contemplation	Not considering change	Locus of control
	Resignation/no control	Health beliefs model
	Denial (re: self relevance)	Motivational interviewing
		Integrated (I-change) model
	Consequences not serious	Social learning theory
Contemplation	Weighing benefits/costs	Theory of reasoned action
		Motivational interviewing
Preparation	Experimenting with change	CBT
		Motivational interviewing
Action	Taking steps to change	Imitation (skinnerian)
		Self-efficacy
		12-step model
		Health action process
Maintenance	Maintaining behavior	Reinforcement (Skinner)
		12-step model
Relapse	Normal part of process	Motivational interviewing
	Feels demoralization	Relational frame theory

routinely double parking and snarling traffic. This also translates to facilitating behavior change: people respond more readily when they see the immediate relevance of behavior changes. Knowledge of a person's social support system and interests can be used to frame their motivation for change.

When seeking to motivate behavior change, it is also important to know how close the patient is to actually undertaking meaningful lifestyle change. When a patient has not considered change, and is not open to change, the patient is considered "**pre-contemplative.**" People can be pre-contemplative about anything from cutting back on alcohol consumption to applying ice after strenuous activity. As a patient works through the process of changing behavior they move through stages of pre-contemplation, contemplation, preparation, action, and maintenance, with an occasional relapse. The steps of applying this model are presented in Figure 14.1 and give the provider a framework to understand the challenges and focus of work needed in each stage. Rollick and Miller's landmark book "Motivational Interviewing" is now in a second edition and provides excellent guidance to those interested in a deeper understanding (Miller and Rollnick 2002).

Motivational interviewing and the stages of change model have been successful in many areas of chronic disease management from substance use disorder, to weight management, to pain (Table 14.2). In addition, these methods are consistent with active application of the Four pillars of medical ethics, i.e. autonomy, beneficence, non-maleficence, and distributive justice, especially autonomy, Chapter 5. In addition, these methods build upon

Pain Medicine at a Glance, First Edition. Beth B. Hogans.
© 2022 John Wiley & Sons Ltd. Published 2022 by John Wiley & Sons Ltd.

Figure 14.1 Action items for each stage of stages of change model.

If **pre-contemplative**
    talk about what patient values to discover what's important to them
    frame the risks and benefits of potential change in terms of the values expressed by the patient
If **contemplative**
    Ask about the commitment to change
    Ask about their confidence to change
  Use information about patients values to boost commitment
    emphasize negatives that are most worrisome
    emphasize benefits that are most valuable
      e.g. teens typically worry about white teeth, middle-aged adults worry more about cancer
  Use brainstorming to find small steps would boost confidence
    Ask about what ideas the patient has or has tried
    Propose some small steps that you think might work well
    Make sure to check back on progress
If in **preparation** stage
    Provide support with specific therapies, e.g. prescriptions
    Provide ideas for substantive positive changes (e.g. quit date)
    Continue to support motivation, e.g. commitment, confidence
    Use affirmation and encouragement
If in **action** stage
    Ask about how the change is going
    Support the patient by addressing side effects, problems
    Suggest ways to avoid challenging situations
If in **maintenance** stage
    Ask about the behavior briefly
    Determine if challenges are present and aid if possible.
If in **relapse**
    Express empathy- 'Change is difficult but change has already begun to take place'
    Develop discrepancy – 'How is this different from your goals?'
    Roll with resistance – stop pushing and reflect on patient's standpoint ('Sounds like it's difficult')
    Support self-efficacy - Encourage patient to take up change once more, e.g. 'I believe you can...'

Table 14.2 Motivational interviewing summary.

Readiness for change
Stages of change model
Commitment
Talk values
Confidence
Talk small steps
Strategies
Express empathy
Develop discrepancy
Roll with resistance
Support self-efficacy

insights into establishing the therapeutic relationship, Chapter 9; socioemotional development, Chapter 13; and the management of affect, Chapter 10.

Shared decision-making is the ultimate stage of the motivational interviewing process. Together, the provider and patient identify **treatment options** that are likely to be effective and well adopted by the patient. Preferably, the treatment plan will incorporate treatments that are active, as well as passive strategies, such as pill-taking, where necessary. An example of a shared decision-making plan for a patient with neuropathic pain is shown in Chapter 16.

Documentation is important to the process of motivational interviewing and shared decision-making. This will help the provider rapidly pick up with the plan when the patient returns for a next visit. This gives both patient and provider a *sense of **accountability** to the treatment planning process*.

Checking in and planning next steps: The shared decision-making process works best when patient and provider are aware of the elements of the plan and can acknowledge successful changes, identify barriers to more effective engagement in treatment choices, and move forward to next steps or identify new strategies.

References

Agarwal, A.K. and Murinson, B.B. (2012). New dimensions in patient-physician interaction: values, autonomy, and medical information in the patient-centered clinical encounter. Rambam Maimonides Medical Journal 3 (3): e0017.

Emanuel, E.J. and Emanuel, L.L. (1992). Four models of the physician-patient relationship. JAMA 267: 2221–2226.

Miller, W.R. and Rollnick, S. (2002). Motivational Interviewing: Preparing People for Change, 2e. New York: Guilford Press.

Prochaska, J.O., DiClemente, C.C., and Norcross, J.C. (1992). In search of how people change. Applications to addictive behaviors. The American Psychologist 47 (9): 1102–1114.

15 Communication and interprofessional teams caring for patients with pain

In both the acute and chronic pain care setting, pain is ideally addressed through **interprofessional collaboration**. In the **emergency room** setting, a patient contacts a variety of personnel and healthcare professions. Everyone needs to be **responsive** to the patient in severe pain and should report observations of uncontrolled pain immediately. Nurses, physicians, and physician assistances must work **collaboratively** to assess pain and develop and implement an integrated pain management approach, Table 15.1. Multi-modal analgesia is a term that used by anesthesiologists to mean "multiple forms of pain-relieving medication". Therefore, terms like comprehensive and integrated are needed to describe the application of pharmacological and non-pharmacological treatments. Although modalities such as cold and warm compresses, bolsters, and bed assignments are clearly in the domain of nursing pain control measures, this does not mean that physicians should not attend to these details and communicate with nursing staff if the patient has needs in these areas. In the same vein, when nurses observe inadequate pharmacological pain control, insufficient diagnostic testing, or unclear diagnostic situations, the communication should raise the issues with the appropriate prescribing provider. **Respectful, timely, and collaborative communication** is the key. It is much easier to elicit cooperation when collaboration is the underlying mode of interaction. At pain meetings, a favorite saying is that *"pain management is as team sport"*. This is a great idea to always keep in mind as you approach the patient with pain.

In **acute care settings** such as emergency rooms, providers work at the same workstation and interact directly and continuously. In other acute care settings, providers come into frequent contact and electronic messaging can facilitate the communication of pain care needs. In this setting, and others, anticipation of pain care needs can help to generate a more satisfactory experience for the patient in pain. Having **protocols** in place to provide comprehensive pain treatments for patients undergoing surgeries or procedures, with checklists, established pain reassessment times, and decision cut-points is helpful to communicate expectations amongst providers and staff. **The Joint Commission (TJC)**, besides mandating pain assessment, has mandated education about pain, and safe implementation of pain treatment practices (Baker 2016). Because pain medicines are more effective when used in the context of **appropriate non-pharmacological**

Table 15.1 Strategies for acute pain care management.

Pain outcomes dashboard
Pain plan-of-care checklist
Coordination of pharmacological and non-pharmacological treatments
Protocol for reporting inadequate pain relief and side effects
In-service education about pain

Table 15.2 Key messages from The Joint Commission about pain.

Pain must be assessed and re-assessed appropriately
Patient risk factors for treatment must be evaluated and mitigated
The healthcare organization must have active engagement in managing pain outcomes and treatment risks
Education about pain is essential

Table 15.3 The Joint Commission: standards for pain care.

"Our foundational standards are quite simple. They are:
• The hospital educates all licensed independent practitioners on assessing and managing pain
• The hospital respects the patient's right to pain management
• The hospital assesses and manages the patient's pain"

treatments, and because the choice of non-pharmacological treatments varies from condition to condition, it is important to utilize **plan of care pathways** where possible, this will allow providers to develop comprehensive treatment approaches and to utilize both non-pharmacological and pharmacological treatments, Tables 15.2 and 15.3. Patients **with co-morbid substance use disorders** may have specific needs regarding pain management in acute care settings. These patients may have **multiple pain-associated conditions**, and when prolonged **opioid exposure** is present, they may have increased sensitivity to pain, i.e. lower pain thresholds, lower pain tolerance, and decreased responsiveness to opioids, i.e. tolerance. Opioids demonstrate remarkable tachyphylaxis so that patients that have been on opioids for even a few weeks may demonstrate decreased pain relief in response to ordinary doses (Chapter 21). This is a context where it is critically important to have solid and positively oriented interprofessional communication (Fishman et al. 2013). The prescribing provider must know if a pain medication once administered is associated with ineffective pain relief or excessive sedation. The provider at the bedside needs to be assured that the reports of pain or sedation will be responded to **promptly and appropriately**.

Multidisciplinary case conferences are one mechanism to promote interprofessional collaboration around pain care. A **hospital pain task force** or committee is another mechanism to provide longer-range **oversite** and systemic solutions to pain management challenges. In reviewing sentinel events for pain hospital wide, it is possible to target education to units or service lines that need additional support or guidance. It is important that pain committees have multiprofessional representation and engagement, Table 15.4.

In the **outpatient setting**, interprofessional engagement can be substantially more challenging to implement. However, as you

Pain Medicine at a Glance, First Edition. Beth B. Hogans.
© 2022 John Wiley & Sons Ltd. Published 2022 by John Wiley & Sons Ltd.

Table 15.4 How to communicate with other providers about pain.

Engage the patient in facilitating communication
Copy providers appropriately
Carefully review and respond to communications from others
Anticipate that all written communications can be read by others
Check to make sure you've understood a problem before responding

Table 15.5 Maintaining an excellent reputation.

Avoid disparaging language
Never write an angry email
Express appreciation for those who have gone above expectations
Interprofessional case conferences are not feasible in all care settings. Make sure to copy the patient's primary care provider so that they are aware of progress and relevant developments
When a family member asks about a patient, involve the patient in the conversation. If the patient cannot participate directly, seek their explicit written permission first before any discussion is held
Nothing is more frustrating for a patient than to be treated as if their problem is not worth addressing. If you cannot figure the problem out, provide a referral to someone who might know what is wrong
Never tell a patient that their x ray looks like that of a 90-year old

Source: Based on Watson (2017).

begin to listen to and respond to patients with pain, you will quickly realize that you don't know everything there is to know about pain. This is where working with skillful allied health providers will come to your advantage. When you are starting out in practice, you may discover that your training did not prepare you for every challenge, this is especially true in pain as very little time is committed to this in medical training especially. One Canadian study found that *veterinarians have seven times more training in pain assessment and management than physicians* (Watt-Watson et al. 2009). A skilled physical therapist may know well conditions not covered in adequate detail in medical school or residency. If you were trained in an allopathic medical school, you may have received a scant three hours of formal training about back pain (Mezei et al. 2011). The spine is a complex bio-engineering miracle tasked with strength, flexibility, and rotational capacity, and stability in all directions. There are many conditions of the spine alone that are not covered in traditional training environments. This is true for each part of the body, from the head to the toes. A skilled **psychiatrist, nurse, physical therapist, occupational therapist, psychologist, pharmacist, podiatrist, acupuncturist, dietician,** and others can all contribute meaningfully to a comprehensive treatment plan. Generally, occupational therapy addresses problems related to hand and arm use, physical therapy (PT) address other physical rehabilitation needs such as walking, standing, balance. It is important to identify physical therapists with special skill sets, e.g. headache therapy, women's health, etc. within your referral network to improve outcomes and provide clear guidance to patients seeking to benefit from PT therapy. It is essentially important to remember that respectful, appreciative, and reciprocal communication is the most important tool in obtaining help for your patients. All of us are professionals, and most are striving towards good professional relationships. Humility is often unexpected and appreciated when warranted. Asking curious questions is often the best way to open a conversation (Watson 2017), Table 15.5.

References

Baker, D.W. (2016). Joint commission statement on pain management. 18 April 2016. https://www.jointcommission.org/joint_commission_statement_on_pain_management/ (accessed 19 December 2017).

Fishman, S.M., Young, H.M., Lucas Arwood, E. et al. (2013). Core competencies for pain management: results of an interprofessional consensus summit. Pain Medicine 14 (7): 971–981.

Mezei, L., Murinson, B.B. et al. (2011). Pain education in North American medical schools. The Journal of Pain 12 (12): 1199–1208.

Watson, L. (2017). Why should we educate for inquisitiveness? In: Intellectual Virtues and Education: Essays in Applied Virtue Epistemology (Routledge Studies in Contemporary Philosophy), 1e (ed. J. Baehr), 38–53. New York: Routledge; (18 June 2017).

Watt-Watson, J., McGillion, M. et al. (2009). A survey of prelicensure pain curricula in health science faculties in Canadian universities. Pain Research & Management 14 (6): 439–444.

This is the most important chapter in the entire book. The most important principle of pain management is: *patients with high self-efficacy have better long-term outcomes.* In practical terms, a pain pill will relieve pain for a few hours, a successful home exercise program will relieve pain for decades (Martinez-Calderon et al. 2017). The challenge is to promote self-efficacy and engage patients in therapies that require a personal investment of time and effort. The stakes are high: thousands have died because it was quicker to prescribe some pain medication that it was to convince a reluctant patient to take on some physical therapy. It might seem quicker and "make the patient happy" but too many quick fixes have led to societal mayhem.

The best pain management plans incorporate pharmacological and non-pharmacological treatments. In acute pain management, the first four letters of RICE-M are nonpharmacological. For diabetic nerve pain, moderate exercise and healthy diet are essential to successful treatment. And for chronic back pain where engagement in relaxation, exercise, stretching, and ergonomics is indispensable. As shown in Figure 16.1, many modalities can be utilized to address pain. This diagram can be used to guide provider and patients in developing comprehensive treatment plans that don't require opioids. Sometimes medication allows for some pain control so that active modalities can be embraced.

Balanced pharmacological therapies are explored in the next chapter and provider-directed non-pharmacological therapies, e.g. physical therapy, clinical psychology, acupuncture, and interventional approaches are covered in several chapters, here we will discuss the potential for selected patient-led nonpharmacological therapies to contribute to successful pain management.

Relaxation and meditation are safe and potentially effective methods to help address the disability, suffering and loss of self-efficacy that accompany chronic pain. It is well established that anticipated acute pain, such as that of childbirth can respond well to meditative and **self-hypnotic approaches** with sufficient advance training. Even with the wide-spread adoption of epidural analgesia for childbirth, training for management of obstetric pain remains popular. The efficacy of **mindfulness based stress reduction meditation** was first demonstrated conclusively in the early 1980s (Kabat-Zinn et al. 1985) and has been promulgated through a variety of channels including seminar training sessions, single encounters as part of a broader educational program about pain self-management, audio media, and retreat programs. **Apps** are now an especially popular option for patients willing to engage in this modality.

Moderate daily exercise is widely unappreciated in chronic pain management however, evidence from literature on fibromyalgia, and arthritis support the use of moderate daily exercise. Daily exercise promotes endogenous pain relief mechanisms that are important to reducing dependence on passive pain-control strategies. Moderate daily exercise should focus on cardiovascular conditioning and strength training.

Home exercise programs (HEP) are tailored strength-building exercises designed for each patient's specific needs. Most physical therapists are highly trained in recognizing contributing factors that establish and perpetuate chronic musculoskeletal problems. Weakness in related muscle groups, poor posture, atrophy of small stabilizing muscle groups, core muscle debilitation, maladaptive neuromuscular patterns all contribute to chronic pain

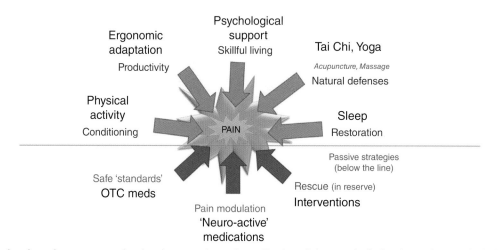

Comprehensive pain treatment: multimodal

Figure 16.1 Comprehensive pain management involves incorporation and coordination of pharmacological and non-pharmacological therapies. The figure below can be shared with patients to prompt discussion and can also serve as a roadmap for clinicians as they assemble a pain management plan for and with their patients.

Given it is not healthy for anyone to rely only on painkillers long-term, I would be interested in trying the following:

Physical therapy	Yoga	Acupuncture
Occupational therapy	Daily walks	Massage
Dance	Ice	Self-massage
Art	Heat packs	TENS
Music	Heating pad	Sleep clinic
Meditation	Psychology	Ergonomics

Figure 16.2 Exploring therapy options: providing patients with prompts and requesting their active input into developing the treatment plan is a way to reinvigorate discussion and forward momentum. Below is a page that can be shared with patients to prompt discussion about non-pharmacological options of interest. **See Chapter 25 for convincing evidence about the effectiveness of non-pharmacological therapies.**

and disability. Physical therapists will often adjust the exercise programs to a patient's ability to participate and their comfort level, and many are experts in motivation! An additional bonus is that an accomplished physical therapist will often identify a previously unsuspected diagnosis and aid in developing a more effective treatment plan. For some patients, **fear of pain** will prevent them from attending physical therapy when first recommended. It is important to **explore barriers** and interfering **misbeliefs** that are preventing engagement. It is also essential to **ask about PT and HEP** compliance at follow up visits. In some cases, an interventional pain treatment may get pain under immediate control, however, remind patients that the temporary relief usually experienced after any kind of pain injection is really an opportunity to pursue a more permanent improvement through focused exercise and conditioning.

Sleep is indispensable to pain control. There is a yin-and-yang relationship between sleep and pain. Poor sleep leads to more pain and more pain leads to worse sleep. **Poor sleep and pain are mutually-perpetuating** (Smith and Haythornthwaite 2004). More detail about this is found in Chapter 25.

Patients have **strong beliefs** about what types of therapies work best for them, and regional and cultural factors pertain; this is why each patient needs a tailored pain treatment plan. One way to

explore non-pharmacological therapies is to provide a list of options and ask what kinds of therapy a patient is most interested in pursuing, Figure 16.2. It is important to be aware of **ethnic and cultural differences** and preferences in nonpharmacological therapies. Recent studies indicate that ethnic groups may demonstrate increase utilization of certain **complementary and alternative medicine (CAM)** modalities. For example, African-Americans have been found to demonstrate high rates of utilizing prayer, herbal remedies, and relaxation (Brown et al. 2007). Hispanic populations have been found to display high rates of utilizing prayer, herbs, and diet (Mikhail et al. 2004). A commonality is that most populations have high interest in CAM modalities especially **diets and supplements**. It is important to know population trends but to recognize that each patient is a unique person and **individual and cultural values** must both be appraised and incorporated into treatment for results to be optimal.

In summary, coordinated comprehensive pain management involves incorporating multiple pharmacological and non-pharmacological approaches with knowledge of selecting treatments likely to effective and readily adopted by the patient. A checklist, as in Figure 16.2, can facilitate communication. In the chapters that follow, potential component treatments are explored.

References

Brown, C.M., Barner, J.C., Richards, K.M., and Bohman, T.M. (2007). Patterns of complementary and alternative medicine use in African Americans. Journal of Alternative and Complementary Medicine 13 (7): 751–758.

Kabat-Zinn, J., Lipworth, L., and Burney, R. (1985). The clinical use of mindfulness meditation for the self-regulation of chronic pain. Journal of Behavioral Medicine 8 (2): 163–190.

Martinez-Calderon, J., Zamora-Campos, C., Navarro-Ledesma, S., and Luque-Suarez, A. (2017). The role of self-efficacy on the prognosis of chronic musculoskeletal pain: a systematic review. The Journal of Pain pii: S1526-5900(17)30699-5.

Mikhail, N., Wali, S., and Ziment, I. (2004). Use of alternative medicine among Hispanics. Journal of Alternative and Complementary Medicine 10 (5): 851–859.

Smith, M.T. and Haythornthwaite, J.A. (2004). How do sleep disturbance and chronic pain inter-relate? Insights from the longitudinal and cognitive-behavioral clinical trials literature. Sleep Medicine Reviews 8 (2): 119–132.

17 Basic considerations for pharmacological therapy – balancing mechanisms of drugs and disease

Rational pharmacotherapy for pain. Pharmacotherapy for pain conditions is based on several principles that allow the development of a medication treatment strategy that will **maximize patient outcomes while limiting side effects**. The principles include: (i) combining medications from complementary classes where appropriate, (ii) not combining medications from within the same class unless absolutely necessary, (iii) tailored agent selection. For example, patients must choose between naproxen and ibuprofen but not take both at the same time. Educating patients about treatment modes of action, i.e. short-acting vs. induction therapy (neuromodulating agents), **black box warnings**, contraindications, potential side effects, and approaches to **cessation or weaning** is essential. In this chapter, a mechanism-based approach to pain medication selection is explained in detail, along with approaches to managing risks, side effects, and treatment failures.

Matching basic mechanism to therapeutic class. As described in Chapter 3, there are three main pain mechanisms: nociceptive, inflammatory, and neuropathic. Inflammatory pain is distinguished by action of an inflammatory mediator on the sensory nervous system to enhance pain signaling and recruit non-painful afferents into pain signaling. Neuropathic pain is distinguished by pain that arises from disease or dysfunction of the nervous system, this could be detectable with diagnostic tests or may occur at the molecular level, either case presenting substantive clinical challenges (Merskey 2007). **The benefit of understanding the major pain mechanism or mechanisms at work is that specific medications work best for each of these mechanisms** (Figure 17.1). Nociceptive pain, when mild, e.g., sprains and strains, usually responds to OTC analgesia. Severe nociceptive pain, as in the setting of trauma or surgery, may require nerve blocks, local anesthetics, or opioids. Inflammatory pain usually responds well to NSAIDs or occasionally corticosteroids but when severe may require the use of disease-modifying therapy, or when present in those with serious comorbid illness or risks for heart attack or stroke, may necessitate other approaches to treatment. Neuropathic pain is not responsive to standard non-opioid analgesia and often requires prescription neuromodulating agents such as gabapentinoids, other anticonvulsants, or pain-active antidepressants. When pain is due to more than one major mechanism, e.g. back injury with radiculopathy which can produce nociceptive, inflammatory, and neuropathic pain, it is ideal to implement multiple therapies to address the various components of pain.

Remaining patient-centered. On the technical level, being patient-centered means that pain medications are chosen with consideration for the patient's **co-morbid conditions, other medications,** and **individual vulnerabilities**. For example, a patient who takes aspirin daily for prevention of MI or stroke should use

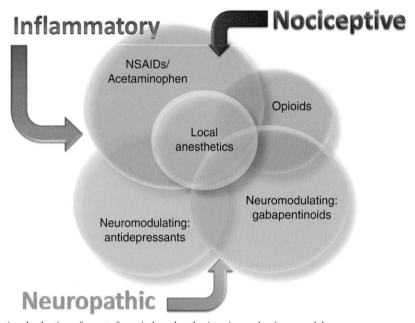

Figure 17.1 Schematic for rational selection of agents for pain based on basic pain mechanisms model.

Pain Medicine at a Glance, First Edition. Beth B. Hogans.
© 2022 John Wiley & Sons Ltd. Published 2022 by John Wiley & Sons Ltd.

Pain type	Non-pharmacological treatements	Pharmacological treatements
Nociceptive	Cold or cooling Rubbing (counter irritant) Distraction	NSAIDs Local anesthetics Opioids (severe+acute)
Inflammatory	Warmth (heating pad, epsom salts), or cooling Gentle exercise PT: Strengthening Stretching, bracing	NSAIDs Acetaminophen* (non anti-inflammatory) Disease modifiers Minimize opioid use
Neuropathic	Distraction Self-management CBT/ACT PT, empathetic support	Pain-active antidepress. Pain-active anticonvuls Local anesthetics Minimize opioid use

Figure 17.2 Treatment according to pain type, summary notes.

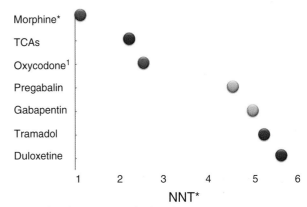

Figure 17.3 Efficacy (NNT) of selected agents.

NSAIDs only rarely. This is because NSAIDs can counteract the anti-platelet effects of aspirin; in clinical trials ibuprofen eliminates the benefits of aspirin (Bally et al. 2017).

On the humanistic level, remaining patient-centered means being aware of the impact of medication choice on lifestyle (Murinson 2009) (Figure 17.2). Small steps such as offering 90-day prescriptions for longer-term medications e.g., pain-active antidepressants can spare patients frequent pharmacy trips. Consider the impact of procedures and testing on patients who have limited mobility. Is the risk associated with stopping a blood thinner sufficiently offset by the anticipated benefit from a planned surgery or procedure? What are the cognitive effects and are these tolerable?

Having an appropriate follow through plan. As Paracelsus noted, every medicine is also a poison. Given the diversity of human biochemistry, not all medications will work for all patients, and some patients will not tolerate specific medications (Figure 17.3). Although some side effects can be mitigated by a "start low and go slow" approach to introducing new medications. Intolerable side effects, such as leg edema associated with gabapentinoid use, necessitate discontinuation. Provide **callback instructions** for side effects, inform whether medications can safely be stopped abruptly and be prepared to try another agent.

Titrating for efficacy. One of the most common clinical missteps observed in pain clinics is the abandonment of a potentially efficacious agent before a full therapeutic trial has been completed. In treating patients with persistent pain or pain that is sub-acute, it is important to explore the safe dose range of a medication before switching to another agent. For example, if low dose tramadol partially relieves a patient's pain without causing side effects, consider increasing the medication dosage.

Minimizing risks of abuse. Some pain medications are prone to misuse, but this does not pertain to all medications utilized for the treatment of pain. For opioids, it is important to prescribe these medications only to those patients who are **screened** for substance abuse risk and **monitored** for safe medication use, in the setting of clear expectations regarding the **duration of therapy**. The approaches to assessing and mitigating opioid abuse risk are discussed in detail in Chapter 48. A few of the non-opioid pain medications, especially tramadol and gabapentin are sometimes abused and careful attention to precautions when prescribing these medications is necessary. Application of good standard principles of prescribing: the **Right patient**, for the **Right condition**, in the **Right amount**, for the **Right duration**, as well as attention to whether the medications chosen are appropriate for the basic pain mechanisms at work.

In summary, rational pharmacotherapy for pain involves knowing or making an educated proposition regarding the basic pathophysiology of a pain condition, and then selecting medications that are most likely to address the pathophysiological processes associated with that mechanism. You do not always have to know the exact pain condition that a patient is experiencing to begin rational pharmacotherapy: the proposed pain mechanisms, characteristics of the patient, and the clinical setting all play a role in choosing the right medications.

References

Bally, M., Dendukuri, N., Rich, B. et al. (2017). Risk of acute myocardial infarction with NSAIDs in real world use: bayesian meta-analysis of individual patient data. BMJ 357: j1909.

Merskey, H. (2007). The taxonomy of pain. The Medical Clinics of North America 91 (1): 13–20. vii.

Murinson, B.B. (2009). A mechanism-based approach to pain pharmacotherapy: targeting pain modalities for optimal treatment efficacy. In: Current Therapy in Pain (ed. H. Smith), 397–402. Philadelphia, PA: Saunders Elsevier.

18 Over-the-counter analgesia: Non-steroidal anti-inflammatory drugs (NSAIDs) and acetaminophen

Non-steroidal anti-inflammatory drugs (NSAIDs) are the most valuable medications for basic management of mild-to-moderate pain worldwide. These medications are especially effective for nociceptive and inflammatory pain but ineffective against neuropathic pain. **Acetaminophen** is also widely used for relief of mild and mild-moderate pain, it has a distinctive mechanism of action and although antipyretic, lacks anti-inflammatory effects (Figure 18.1). Use is limited by ceiling effects in analgesia. Both NSAIDs and acetaminophen can precipitate fatalities: knowledge and care are necessary when using these drugs.

NSAIDs interfere with **prostaglandin production** by blocking cyclo-oxygenase 1 and 2 (COX1 and COX2). NSAIDs vary in terms of relative potency against COX1 and COX2 with important implications, Table 18.1. The primary problematic NSAID side effect is GI bleeding, due to COX1 inhibition interfering with intrinsic gastroprotective mechanisms. COX2 activity is inducible and important for inflammatory pain signaling and the efficacy of these medications. Unfortunately, some selective COX2 inhibitors, blockbuster pain medications at one time, were associated with myocardial infarction and death. Only one selective COX2 inhibitor remains available in the U.S.: celecoxib. Use of this medication has fallen off and it is now limited to treatment of highly selected patients for short periods. NSAIDs share some of these risks and there is **increased risk for MI** in patients treated with NSAIDs long-term (Bally et al. 2017). For this reason, NSAIDs should be used at the lowest dose possible for the shortest possible period, especially in older patients. Patients with increased risk of CAD should be evaluated continuously for NSAID necessity, and alternative strategies implemented. Patients should be instructed to stop treatment and seek medical attention for symptoms of GI

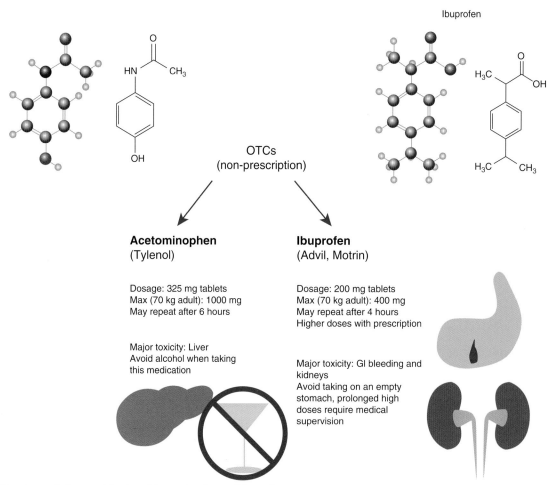

Ibuprofen

OTCs
(non-prescription)

Acetominophen
(Tylenol)

Dosage: 325 mg tablets
Max (70 kg adult): 1000 mg
May repeat after 6 hours

Major toxicity: Liver
Avoid alcohol when taking
this medication

Ibuprofen
(Advil, Motrin)

Dosage: 200 mg tablets
Max (70 kg adult): 400 mg
May repeat after 4 hours
Higher doses with prescription

Major toxicity: GI bleeding and
kidneys
Avoid taking on an empty
stomach, prolonged high
doses require medical
supervision

Figure 18.1 Structure and pharmacokinetics of Acetaminophen and Ibuprofen.

Pain Medicine at a Glance, First Edition. Beth B. Hogans.
© 2022 John Wiley & Sons Ltd. Published 2022 by John Wiley & Sons Ltd.

Table 18.1 Selected NSAIDs and relative potency for COX1 and COX2.

NSAID	COX1 μM	COX2 μM	COX1/COX2	Half-life	Comments
Aspirin	0.3	50	0.006	4 h	COX1 selective
Ibuprofen	1	15	0.067	4 h	Most widely used NSAID
Naproxen	2.2	1.3	1.69	11 h	Longer-acting NSAID
Diflofenac	0.5	0.35	1.43	6 h	Higher potency
Etodolac	>100	53	>1.9	6–7 h	High COX2 selectivity (Kato et al. 2001)
Meloxicam	37	6.1	6.1	20 h	High COX2 selectivity (Kato et al. 2001)
Celocoxib	1.2	0.34	3.53	6 h	COX2 selective agent
Acetaminophen	2.7	20	N/A	4 h	Anti-pyretic, not anti-inflammatory

bleeding, chest pain, shortness of breath, stroke, or altered urination. Renal injury is associated with chronic NSAID use and some NSAIDs cause blood pressure elevations which may in part account for cardiac and renal effects. Some preclinical evidence suggests that NSAIDs impede skeletal healing and some surgeons may avoid NSAIDs post-operatively.

Despite these limitations, NSAIDs reduce episodic nociceptive or inflammatory pain. For occasional tension headache, ibuprofen is often completely effective. When taken at the first sign of headache, **ibuprofen** is as effective as some triptan medications in stopping **migraines** (Xu et al. 2016). The importance of early medication administration in managing migraine cannot be over-emphasized, sometimes the most effective intervention can be to carry fast-acting ibuprofen and a water bottle everywhere. Ibuprofen, **naproxen** and other NSAIDs are highly effective for ordinary sprains and strains, post-exertional muscle pain, and moderate osteoarthritis.

It is essential to observe dosage limits with some adjustments for patient body mass. While a 50-kg person should not exceed 400 mg ibuprofen, larger people may need higher doses to obtain relief. Prescription strength ibuprofen is available in 600 and 800 mg formulations. The dosing interval increases as the dose increases so that 400 mg may be given every four hours, 600 mg every six hours, and 800 mg every eight hours.

Recent meta-analysis indicates that "salted" formulations of ibuprofen are associated with **relief that is faster, more durable, and more effective** overall (Moore et al. 2014). These formulations are not "standard" in the U.S. but are available as **ibuprofen sodium** and ibuprofen acetate in selected preparations. At present, this looks like great news for patients seeking faster, more effective pain relief.

Over the counter NSAIDs include naproxen which has important advantages, including a longer duration of action such that the tablets are to be taken every 12 hours. In addition, there is some evidence that the cardiac risks, associated with several NSAIDs, may be somewhat lower. It is important that patients observe stated limits on dosage, not infrequently patients will try taking more naproxen than recommended. Patients should be warned that NSAIDs in excess can lead to cardiac events including MI and death, as well as renal failure, and potentially fatal GI bleeding.

Some NSAIDs are available only be prescription, including NSAID medications with once daily dosing regimens and COX2 selectivity, e.g. meloxicam, etodolac.

Acetaminophen has a distinctive mechanism of action and while not useful as an anti-inflammatory medication, it can reduce fever. Acetaminophen acts centrally, inhibiting Cyclo-oxygenase 3 (**COX3**) as well as COX1 and COX2 less potently. Side effects are distinctive; the primary toxicity is for liver. Acetaminophen is metabolized in the liver and reactive oxygen species arise that can destroy liver parenchyma. This is a dose-dependent effect that limits that maximum tolerable dosage of acetaminophen. Current FDA recommendations are that **acetaminophen** from all sources should **not exceed 3000 mg daily**. Vigilance is needed because acetaminophen is compounded into over-the-counter preparations and combined with opioids and other pain relievers. Prescribing providers should caution patients that daily total dosage of acetaminophen cannot exceed 3000mg. It is important to counsel patients who consume alcohol to refrain from or decrease alcohol consumption during acetaminophen treatment. The patients who were most vulnerable to acetaminophen toxicity were those with baseline liver compromise or alcohol consumption. Acetaminophen, in moderation can be safely combined with most other pain-active medications and due to a distinctive mechanism of action can provide additional pain relief even to patients with fairly complex medical regimens.

Finally, while acetaminophen is generally safe **in pregnancy, NSAIDs should be avoided**, especially in the third trimester.

In summary, over-the-counter standard analgesics and prescription NSAIDs are valuable for pharmacological management of pain. It is important for prescribers to observe precautions and monitor for side effects.

References

Bally, M., Dendukuri, N., Rich, B. et al. (2017). Risk of acute myocardial infarction with NSAIDs in real world use: bayesian meta-analysis of individual patient data. BMJ 357: j1909.

Kato, M., Nishida, S., Kitasato, H. et al. (2001). Cyclooxygenase-1 and cyclooxygenase-2 selectivity of non-steroidal anti-inflammatory drugs: investigation using human peripheral monocytes. The Journal of Pharmacy and Pharmacology 53 (12): 1679–1685.

Moore, R.A., Derry, S., Straube, S. et al. (2014). Faster, higher, stronger? Evidence for formulation and efficacy for ibuprofen in acute pain. Pain 155 (1): 14–21.

Xu, H., Han, W., Wang, J., and Li, M. (2016). Network meta-analysis of migraine disorder treatment by NSAIDs and triptans. The Journal of Headache and Pain 17 (1): 113.

19 Neuromodulating agents: pain-active anti-depressants and anti-convulsants

Multiple medications that are not traditional analgesics possess proven efficacy against persistent pain (Figure 19.1). As a group, these pain-active medications act through neuromodulating mechanisms. They are useful for the treatment of neuropathic pain, which is often (i) persistent over years, (ii) generally unresponsive to over-the-counter analgesia, and (iii) difficult to manage otherwise (Cruccu and Truini 2017). Most neuro-modulating agents, except pregabalin, were not initially developed for pain, although now, several have FDA indications for painful conditions.

Pain-active antidepressants include multiple tricyclic antidepressants (TCA's) and some newer anti-depressants, with noradrenergic activity. **Blackbox suicidality warnings pertain to all pain-active antidepressants** (Table 19.1). These SNRIs (selective serotonin and norepinephrine reuptake inhibitors) as a group are effective against pain to some degree. Although characterized by substantive side effects, such as dry mouth and genitourinary dysfunction, TCA's have very high rates of efficacy with the "number needed to treat" (NNT (glossary)) for these agents ranging from 2 to 3 in clinical trials. Newer antidepressants such as duloxetine (Cymbalta) and venlafaxine (Effexor) have a higher NNT than do TCAs. However, the newer antidepressants demonstrate milder side effect profiles.

Amitriptyline is the **prototypical pain-active antidepressant**. Although use is constrained by **prominent cholinergic** side effects, it is highly effective in the proper setting. Because amitriptyline causes sedation, dry mouth (xerostomia), urinary delay, constipation, and sexual dysfunction, patients must be counseled about the side effects. Fortunately, the sedating effects of amitriptyline can be beneficial in those patients with pain at night. Many patients with neuropathic or persistent pain find that pain is more pronounced at nighttime, interfering with both sleep onset and persistence. Amitriptyline induces a strong sense of sleepiness and relieves neuropathic pain when taken consistently. Patients should be warned not to take amitriptyline before driving. The drying of oral mucosa promotes tooth decay and patients should be warned to increase dental hygiene and hydrate. In most patients, it is best to start amitriptyline at a low dose taken before bedtime. 10 mg is a good starting dose for many patients. For amitriptyline and all the TCA's, it is **recommended** that **patients over 40 years undergo a screening EKG** and that treatment not given to those with **QT prolongation. Nortriptyline** is another pain-active antidepressant. It essentially acts like a slow-release amitriptyline. It is not associated with the same profound sedation as amitriptyline, although constipation and urinary delay are frequently cited side effects. The cautions for patients are similar and EKG prior to treatment initiation is recommended for those over age 40. Desipramine is a third TCA; the side effect profile is distinct from that for amitriptyline and nortriptyline. It is not sedating which many patients appreciate, however it produces tachycardia and this can be a treatment-limiting effect. Newer pain-active antidepressants include venlafaxine (Effexor) and duloxetine (Cymbalta); milnacipran (Savella) is used in Europe as an antidepressant but in the U.S. it has FDA approval for FM. **Venlafaxine** is associated with primarily neurocognitive effects but serotonin syndrome has been reported and

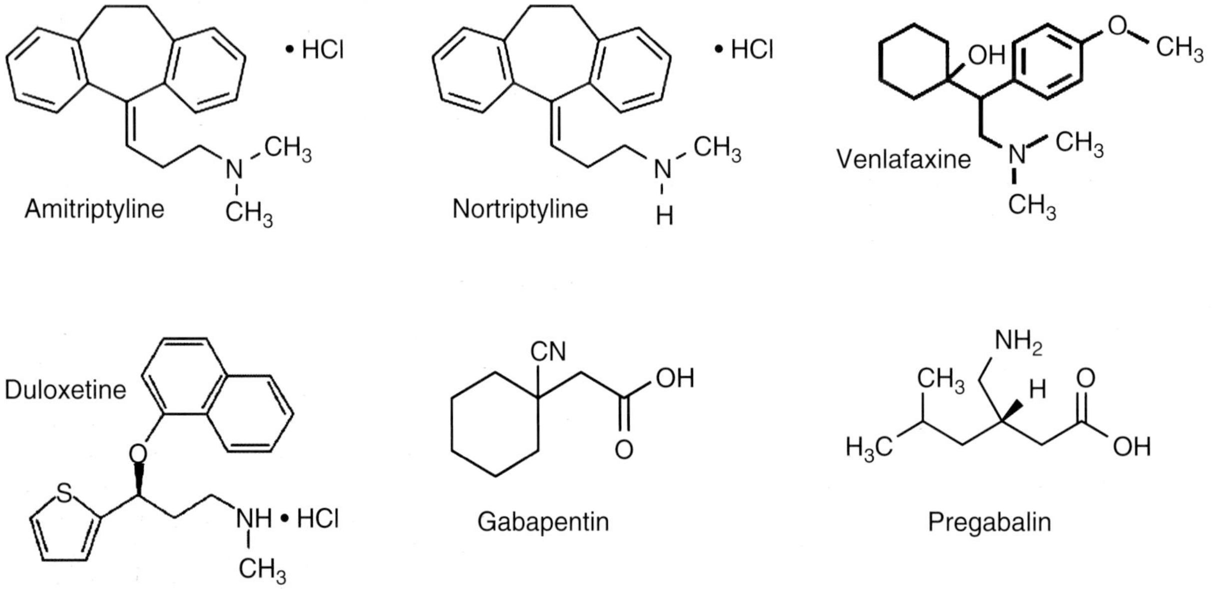

Figure 19.1 Structure of selected neuromodulating agents.

Pain Medicine at a Glance, First Edition. Beth B. Hogans.
© 2022 John Wiley & Sons Ltd. Published 2022 by John Wiley & Sons Ltd.

Table 19.1 Selected features of pain-active neuromodulating agents: anti-depressants and gabapentinoids.

Medication	Trade name	Half-life	Mechanistic features	Efficacy features	Side effects	Cost
amitriptyline	Elavil	13 h	TCA SNRI	Must be taken daily for weeks to work	Strongly sedating drying, cholinergic, SI[a]	$
nortriptyline	Pamelor	26 h	TCA-SNRI	Must be taken daily for weeks to work	Some cholinergic effects, SI[a]	$
desipraimine	Norpramin	15 h	TCA-SNRI	Must be taken daily for weeks to work	Tachycardia, non-sedating, SI[a]	$
venlafaxine	Effexor	5 h IR 10 hER	SNRI	Must be taken daily for weeks to work	Increases HBP, SI[a]	$
duloxetine	Cymbalta	12 h	SNRI	Must be taken daily for weeks to work FDA approved for: CLBP	Irritability, SI[a]	$$
gabapentin	Neurontin	6 h	GABA analogue	FDA approved for: PHN	Dizziness, cognitive effects	$'
pregabalin	Lyrica	6.3 h	GABA analogue	FDA approved for: FM, DPN, SCI-pain, PHN	Ankle edema, cognitive	$$$

[a]All pain-active antidepressants carry blackbox warnings for suicidal ideation. The TCAs (tricyclic-antidepressants) are not appropriate for patients with cardiac conditions and an EKG should be checked for Q-T prolongation in patients over 40, Q-T prolongation at baseline is a contraindication for TCAs. TCAs and venlafaxine are not FDA approved for pain indications however peer-reviewed RCT clinical evidence for pain efficacy is extensive.

serotinergic drug-drug interactions can be prominent. Patients with high blood pressure are not appropriate for venlafaxine (Effexor). **Duloxetine** (Cymbalta) was initially approved as an antidepressant but now holds FDA approval for multiple pain-associated conditions: chronic musculoskeletal pain, fibromyalgia, and diabetic peripheral neuropathy.

Pain-active anti-convulsants historically included phenytoin, carbamazepine, and valproic acid, although with the relatively high efficacy of gabapentinoids (gabapentin and pregabalin) the use of a broader range of anti-convulsants has declined. Certain drugs are still used in selected settings, for example **carbamazepine** remains a first-line therapy for **trigeminal neuralgia**; **topiramate** is widely used for the prophylaxis of **migraine** headache and selectively used for persistent pain in other settings; and lamotrigine has clinically proven efficacy against HIV neuropathy, but not other forms of painful neuropathy. The **gabapentinoids** have played an instrumental role in overturning the therapeutic nihilism that previously characterized the management of diabetic neuropathy. With the introduction of gabapentin in the 1990s, physicians had an agent that was generally safe, well-tolerated, and associated with very few interactions. Well tolerated by most people, **gabapentin** does not carry the risks of dangerous idiosyncratic side effects that characterize most other anticonvulsants. Dosing can begin at 100 mg at bedtime for older patients, or 300 mg at bedtime for younger patients. The most prominent side effects include some mild sedation, disequilibrium, and cognitive interference, it is not uncommon for patients to report difficulty with multitasking. More recently, **pregabalin** has been approved for the treatment of neuropathic pain (Shanthanna et al. 2017). Related chemically to gabapentin, pregabalin has similar effects in terms of reducing pain intensity while not completely eliminating pain altogether. Also

generally well tolerated, the side effect profile is somewhat different, including some cognitive interference and ankle edema, sometimes necessitating treatment cessation. Gabapentinoids act via Alpha-2-delta blockade of pre-synaptic terminals and potentially other mechanisms. Gabapentinoids have renal excretion and must be adjusted in renally impaired patients. Interestingly, pregabalin was observed to produce mild euphoria in some people, this effect is not widely observed but it is important to be aware that pregabalin can have psychogenic effects.

In using the neuromodulating agents, it is important to recognize that **chronic treatment is intended**. While these agents are not associated with SUD as are the opioids, there is a potential for **metabolic interactions**, especially in patients with **renal failure** and for some agents with **hepatic disease**. Dosage adjustments are often required in older patients: for example, gabapentinoid dosing is lower and TCAs should be avoided altogether.

In summary, neuromodulating agents are pain-active medications that are not traditional analgesics. Typically requiring continuous dosing to attain the intended treatment benefits, appropriately selected patients find that neuromodulating agents are an important part of managing chronic pain.

References

Cruccu, G. and Truini, A. (2017). A review of neuropathic pain: from guidelines to clinical practice. Pain and therapy 6 (Suppl 1): 35–42.

Shanthanna, H., Gilron, I., Rajarathinam, M. et al. (2017). Benefits and safety of gabapentinoids in chronic low back pain: A systematic review and meta-analysis of randomized controlled trials. PLoS Medicine 14 (8): e1002369.

Pictographic representations of the **opium poppy** dating to 1550 B.C.E. show that opioid use dates back **3 millennia (Figure** 20.1). Problems with opioids are also known throughout recorded history. A dramatic upswing in opioid utilization after the **U.S. Civil War** led to chilling reports of deaths and deprivation resulting from **patent medicines** at the start of the twentieth Century (Adams 2013). Precipitated by unscrupulous manufacturers who adjured responsibility for ensuing addiction and ignored ghastly consequences of tainted preparations, the patent medicine crisis led to important safety reforms. In large measure driven by opioid and coca dependence, federal legislation spawned the modern-day **U.S. Food and Drug Administration**.

Decades passed and despite the bitter lessons of drug abuse following the **Vietnam War** and rampant drug experimentation of the 1970s, societal defenses against widespread drug use attenuated and were labeled retrogressive. Changes in healthcare and medical education created circumstances in which cautious attitudes toward prescribing opioids were viewed as outmoded and early trends in patient-centered medicine gave rise to notion that **chronic opioid treatment** could be easily negotiated with patients and high doses would relieve pain and restore function. Opioid prescribing began to increase in the late 1980s (Wisconsin Pain and Policy Study Group (PPSG) 2017). Pharmaceutical companies developed massive capacity for producing high purity opioids under pristine manufacturing conditions. Safety seemed assured. In the late 1990s prescribing of opioids further escalated (Figure 20.2).

Many underestimated the potential for opioid addiction as well as the willingness of everyone involved to cut corners. In the early 2000s it was clear that unintentional drug overdose deaths were skyrocketing, by 2007 the rate was nine times that of 30 years earlier. As government agencies sounded the alarm, regulations changed and were reinterpreted (Rudd et al. 2016). Prescribing

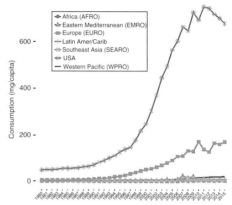

Figure 20.2 Consumption of opioids in the U.S. compared with other global regions, 1980–2015. Sources: International Narcotics Control Board; World health Organization poulation data By: Pain & policy studies group, University of University of Wisconsin WHO Colaborating center, 2017.

levels slowed in 2006 and dropped beginning in 2011, but thousands were already addicted. Some turned to illegal opioids, principally heroin, which had become far less expensive due to advances in technology and new importation patterns. In 2015, suppliers began substituting fentanyl and carfentenil in place of heroin, and people began dying in record numbers from overdose. A crisis was recognized 20 years late.

The fundamental point is that people often seek pain relief from their healthcare providers. Providers, pressed for time and pressured to choose less costly treatments, may not recognize the potential harm of options at their disposal unless properly educated. By reading this book and learning more about pain, you are taking important steps toward preventing harms due to pain treatment as well as undertreatment.

There are settings in which opioid prescribing is appropriate and necessary (Table 20.1). The clearest case for opioids is in **perioperative care**. Much of modern surgery and procedural dentistry would be impossible without opioids. Although nerve block approaches to acute pain management have gained ground in the last decade and are improving surgical and trauma outcomes,

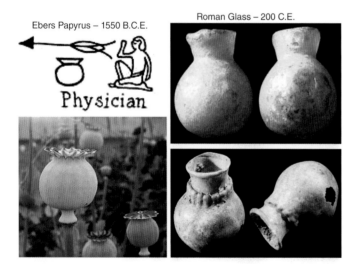

Figure 20.1 Representations of opioids in antiquity.

Table 20.1 Abbreviated guide to appropriate opioid prescribing scenarios.

Scenario	1	2	3
Features	Severe Nociceptive Acute Pain	Chronic Life-limiting Advancing Pain	Temporary Relief Any-old Pain
Mnemonic	SNAP	CLAP	TRAP
Opioids generally appropriate	Yes	Yes	No[a]

[a] Seek a pain specialist consultation for scenarios other than (1) SNAP and (2) CLAP.

When prescribing opioids it is essential to assess risk and manage side effects.

1) Assess the patient's risk of abuse prior to prescribing, even for a short interval
    a. A patient who is 'in recovery' may be destabilized by opioid exposure
    b. A patient who is currently exposed to opioids will need more opioid to obtain pain relief.
2) Assess the patient's profile for adverse effects:
    a. Respiratory compromise greatly increases the risk of opioids. Patients with underlying respiratory conditions, e.g. COPD, Asthma, are at increased risk of death from opioids
    b. Alcohol consumption raises the risk for fatal respiratory suppression
3) Do not co-prescribe benzodiazepines and opioids.
    a. Benzodiazepines potentiate the respiratory suppression effects of opioids
4) Constipation can be so severe with prolonged opioid treatment as to result in death
    a. Provide instructions for managing constipation for courses of 2 days or less.
    b. Provide co-prescribed bowel regimen for courses of 3 days or longer.
5) Nausea, vomiting, and itching are also common side effects of opioids, these may be managed with a reduced dose, ultra-low dose naloxone (in some settings), or coprescribing of antiemetic or antipruritic agents, or choosing a different agent.

Figure 20.3 Opioid precautions.

opioids are remarkably effective in the control of severe acute pain. In the absence of a highly skilled regional anesthesiologist who can block a nerve or place an epidural, opioids offer the best tool for **rapid pain control**. The major limitations are: tachyphylaxis, constipation, respiratory suppression, potential for **death**, and risk of **addiction**.

Before the era of modern analgesia, surgery meant being strapped to a table, having a rag shoved between the teeth, and enduring unbelievable agony. Now, most people can go through procedures involving replacement of vital organs or joints with tolerable amounts of pain. Due to excellence in pain control, people are starting rehabilitation programs the same day as having major surgery, experiencing reduced HPA stress, and lower rates of infection and deep venous thrombosis. We still need opioids in the modern medical world, and we just need to use them safely.

The ability of an analgesic to alleviate pain is called analgesic efficacy. When analgesics are assessed for efficacy, this is measured by the ability of the medicine to reduce pain intensity (McQuay 1999). Often in clinical trials, a medication for chronic pain is considered successful when pain is reduced by three points on a "10 point" scale. When patients undergoing surgery think of a pain medicine working well, they may be thinking in terms "pain relief" which can mean taking severe pain, i.e. 8, 9 or 10 points on a "10 point" scale, and reducing it to no or minimal pain, e.g. 0, 1, or 2 points. This would not be possible for some medicines; however when opioids are used in the setting of acute pain, a patient who is not opioid dependent will obtain nearly complete pain relief from moderate doses of opioids in most cases. For a 70 kg healthy person, this might mean that 5 or 10 mg of oxycodone could relieve post-operative pain for 4–6 hours (Figure 20.3). It is a fundamental truth of modern medicine that opioids are remarkably effective at reducing operative and procedural pain. Unfortunately, patients who are **chronically exposed to opioids have increased pain,** **and lower pain thresholds and less tolerance** (Zahari et al. 2016). Beside the reduction in average pain intensity, the NNT for morphine, given with a dose-to-efficacy protocol, is close to 1, perfect efficacy. The high efficacy of opioids is another central factor that accounts for their durable popularity.

In summary, opioids are particularly useful for severe, nociceptive, acute pain in the perioperative setting. They also continue to be essential for the management of chronic, life-limiting, advancing pain, e.g. terminal cancer pain. Opioids are not ideal for general chronic pain or for the management of general acute pain as the long-term risks outweigh the potential benefits in most patients.

References

Adams, S.H. (2013). The Great American Fraud: A Series of Articles on the Patent Medicine Evil, Reprinted from Collier's Weekly. Project Gutenberg, Release Date: 1 December 2013 [EBook #44325], D Widger (Prod.). https://www.gutenberg.org/files/44325/44325-h/44325-h.htm (accessed 4 July 2017).

McQuay, H.J. (1999). Post-operative analgesia. Best Practice & Research. Clinical Anaesthesiology 13 (3): 465–476.

Pain & Policy Study Group (PPSG) (2017). Opioid Consumption Data Madison, WI 53706: Pain & Policy Studies Group (PPSG). http://www.painpolicy.wisc.edu/opioid-consumption-data (accessed 20 December 2017).

Rudd, R., Aleshire, N., Zibbell, J., and Gladden, M. (2016). Increases in drug and opioid overdose deaths — United States, 2000–2014. MMWR 64 (50): 1378–1382.

Zahari, Z. et al. (2016). Comparison of pain tolerance between opioid dependent patients on methadone maintenance therapy (MMT) and opioid naive individuals. Journal of Pharmacy & Pharmaceutical Sciences (www.cspsCanada.org) 19 (1): 127–136.

21 Opioids – the details: equianalgesia and safe use

Opioids are central to the management of severe acute pain in the post-operative period as well as in advanced cancer pain treatment. Due to the risks associated with opioids, it is important to be mindful of safe use principles, side effects, and toxicities discussed here (Volkow 2014) (Table 21.1). Equianalgesia is especially important with opioids, due to tolerance and some degree of tachyphylaxis. Patients on chronic opioid treatment for pain may require opioid rotation, and when patients are converting from parenteral to oral medication regimens post-operatively, in these contexts it is important to be able to perform opioid conversions to produce equianalgesia.

Equianalgesia. The observation that opioids can often be interchangeably used for the treatment of pain, equianalgesia references other opioids to the potency of morphine against pain. Morphine is the prototypical opioid, and it has a relative potency of 1. Other opioids are gauged relative to morphine, Table 21.2. Fentanyl, for example is much more potent, so that 1 mg of fentanyl will provide analgesia equivalent to 50–200 mg of morphine or 50–200 MME (morphine milligram equivalents) (in naïve patients). For this reason, 1 mg of fentanyl is considered to represent 50–200 morphine equivalents. This is useful when considering opioid consumption on a population basis but may be somewhat different on an individual basis. For more on opioid rotation, see Chapter 47.

Safe opioid use in the acute care setting. When planning a transition from inpatient perioperative pain management to outpatient post-operative pain management, first consider the daily requirement of the patient in the first stages after surgery, and then anticipate the natural course of pain resolution. Many, if not most surgeries invoke **strong nociceptive pain** initially but will demonstrate a resolution of intense pain over the 3–5 days post-op (CDC 2017). Exceptions to this general rule are surgeries that involve extensive work on bone such as multi-level spine surgery, extensive bone work in the pelvis, and some poly-trauma situations.

Table 21.1 The basic principles of safe opioid use are embodied in the CDC and JC guidelines.

Use opioids for the shortest possible time
Limit opioids to the lowest effective dose
Combine opioids with other nonpharmacological and non-opioid treatments
Implement a comprehensive pain treatment plan
Counsel patients about opioid risks including possible death and addiction
Test patients for treatment compliance
Test patients for illicit substance use that may impact opioid safety
Assess for pulmonary disease and risks prior to opioid initiation
Ensure that patients with compromised respiratory function have limited exposure to opioids
Do not combine opioids and benzodiazepines unless expert consultation indicates this is appropriate
Do not provide opioids if they will be combined with alcohol
Advise patients not to drive or operate heavy machinery during treatment with opioids

Table 21.2 Opioid potency relative to morphine, and receptor subtype activation, oral administration.

Drug	"Potency" (relative)	Route	Binding and activation
Morphine	1	p.o.	MOR 1.2 nM DOR 217 nM KOR 26.9 nM
Oxycodone	1.5	p.o.	MOR 18 nM DOR 958 nM KOR 677 nM
Fentanyl	50–200	Trans-dermal	MOR 0.7 nM DOR 153 nM KOR 85 nM
Hydromorphone	4	p.o.	MOR 0.28 nM DOR 38 nM KOR 2.8 nM
Hydromorphone	20	i.v.	
Methadone	3–4 (acute)	p.o.	MOR 5.6 nM DOR 1000 nM KOR 1000 nM
Carfentanil (non-human agent)	10 000-100 000	N/A	

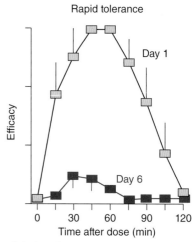

Figure 21.1 Preclinical studies show that there can be very rapid tolerance to morphine analgesic effects. In experimental settings, mice given daily morphine demonstrate marked reductions in relief from pain (behavior) after five days of daily morphine, i.e. morphine on Day 6 compared to Day 1 produces less than 10% of the pain-relieving effect (Ueda and Ueda 2009). Source: Adapted from Ueda and Ueda 2009.

Unless the pain is exceptional or known to be long-lasting, prescription pain medicine supplies provided to patients should be limited to reflect the anticipated short period of severe post-surgical pain. Adherence to safe opioid prescribing principles is essential, Figure 21.1.

Pain Medicine at a Glance, First Edition. Beth B. Hogans.
© 2022 John Wiley & Sons Ltd. Published 2022 by John Wiley & Sons Ltd.

Table 21.3 Opioid receptor types and actions.

Type	Protypical ligand	Primary actions
μ_1	Most opioids	supraspinal analgesia, euphoria, confusion, dizziness, nausea
μ_2	Morphine	resp. suppression, CV and GI and GU effects
δ	Enkephalin	spinal analgesia
κ	Dynorphin	spinal analgesia, sedation, miosis, psychomimetic, dysphoria, endorphin feedback inhibition
σ	(+)-NANM	psychomimetic effects

Many patients will experience profound constipation with opioids relieved only when able to stop opioid analgesia in the first days after surgery. Severe constipation can develop with only 2–3 days of opioids, it is important to maintain hydration, utilize bowel stimulants, and encourage opioid tapering and opioid-sparing pain regimens. In extreme cases, constipation evolves into **obstipation** and may **be life-threatening** leading to sepsis, bowel perforation, or bacteremia. To some extent, the side effect profile of specific opioids is a reflect of opioid subtypes which bind the drugs and mediate their action, Table 21.3.

Respiratory suppression is a serious and **life-threatening** side effect of opioids that requires careful **assessment** of potential **pulmonary compromise before opioids** are started or continued (The Joint Commission (TJC) 2012). Co-prescription with benzodiazepines should be avoided unless active expert involvement of certified pain medicine experts and psychiatry necessitates such dual agent treatment.

Finally, opioids demonstrate some degree of tachyphylaxis meaning that the pain-relieving effects of opioids rapidly diminish with continued dosing. In preclinical studies, continuous dosing of opioids on a daily basis leads to a state of diminished opioid responsiveness such that the analgesia resulting from a fixed dose of morphine on day 7 is 1/10th that observed on day 1. (Ueda and Ueda 2009) **Opioid tachyphylaxis** means that *increasing doses of opioids would be required to maintain equianalgesia* from one week to the next, escalating doses of opioids were prevalent in the 1990s and lead to people were receiving upwards of 300 MmEq daily. This is very hazardous because there is strong clinical evidence that mortality increases as daily opioids doses increase, most of this mortality is related to respiratory failure.

For many years, opioids were very popular for the management of acute and chronic pain. Beginning in 2016, the CDC issued guidelines for the use of opioids in pain management which dramatically called into question the perception that opioids could be safely "titrated to efficacy" in a wide array of patients. In fact, the CDC called on providers to limit opioid prescriptions to short periods of time for most conditions, and to limit the total milligram amounts given each day (CDC 2017). Providers were instructed to avoid prescribing more than 90 mg daily (morphine equivalents) and to know that **opioids aren't routine for chronic pain** and are not first line therapy for chronic pain. At the peak of the opioid prescribing in 2011, over 219 million prescriptions were written. Total consumption of prescribed opioids, other than methadone, in the U.S. reached 555 mg per person annually, meaning that if an opioid naïve person needs 10 mg of morphine to relieve bone pain for six hours (assuming a broken bone hurts severely for three days), this is enough morphine for every person to sustain four major bone fractures a year. This is in counter-poise with evidence that nearly half of patients with advanced and terminal cancer have poorly controlled pain, and with the evidence that shows that there are persistent disparities in access to pain medications, even in the U.S. a country which consumes a large portion of the global opioid supply (Pain and Policy Study Group (PPSG) 2017).

In summary, opioids remain essential for the control of severe peri-operative pain and advanced cancer pain. Particular characteristics and hazards of opioids mean that additional knowledge is necessary for safe use.

References

CDC (2017). Guideline for prescribing opioids for chronic pain. https://www.cdc.gov/drugoverdose/pdf/guidelines_factsheet-a.pdf (accessed 20 December 2017).

Galligan, J.J. and Akbarali, H.I. (2014). Molecular physiology of enteric opioid receptors. American Journal of Gastroenterology Supplements 2 (1): 17–21.

Green, C.R. and Hart-Johnson, T. (2012). The association between race and neighborhood socioeconomic status in younger Black and White adults with chronic pain. The Journal of Pain 13 (2): 176–186.

Kapitzke, D., Vetter, I., and Cabot, P.J. (2005). Endogenous opioid analgesia in peripheral tissues and the clinical implications for pain control. Therapeutics and Clinical Risk Management 1 (4): 279–297.

Pain and Policy Study Group (PPSG) (2017). Morphine Equivalence. University of Wisconsin-Madison http://www.painpolicy.wisc.edu/sites/www.painpolicy.wisc.edu/files/country_files/morphine_equivalence/unitedstatesofamerica_me_methadone.pdf (accessed 20 December 2017).

The Joint Commission (TJC) (2012). Safe use of opioids in hospitals. The Joint Commission Sentinel Event Alert 49, 8 August 2012.

Ueda, H. and Ueda, M. (2009). Mechanisms underlying morphine analgesic tolerance and dependence. Frontiers in Bioscience 14: 5260–5272.

Volkow, ND (Presenter) (2014). America's addiction to opioids: heroin and prescription drug abuse. 14 May 2014 Senate Caucus on International Narcotics Control. https://www.drugabuse.gov/about-nida/legislative-activities/testimony-to-congress/2016/americas-addiction-to-opioids-heroin-prescription-drug-abuse.

22 Opioids – advanced practice – alternative delivery routes: IV, PCA, epidural

Opioids can be delivered through a variety of routes when appropriate (Figure 22.1). In the **inpatient setting**, options include IV, and epidural routes combined with patient-controlled analgesia (PCA) administration. In the **outpatient setting**: transdermal and intrathecal routes may pertain. In **palliative care settings**: buccal, sublingual, rectal and subcutaneous administration may be used. Implantable delivery devices, e.g. intrathecal delivery, are limited to pain specialist referral at present. Intranasal use is a specialty application with substantive risks.

Intravenous. IV delivery of opioids is common practice. It is important to recognize that the onset of opioids given IV is rapid and may be associated with respiratory suppression and death. The Joint Commission has mandated pain assessment and management but has also mandated evaluation of patients for respiratory fitness prior to opioid pain management, Chapter 21. **PCA** is very popular with

patients and providers since the advent of sophisticated programmable pumps and can be utilized with IV or epidural delivery systems. Patients are provided with a basal level of opioid, which may be zero, and this is supplemented with additional dose or doses when the patient presses a button. It is felt that over-sedation is avoided because sleepy patients will not be able to press the button, however, family members at the bedside need to be educated about proper use of the PCA. If the patient requires opioid pain management at the time of hospital discharge, it is necessary to convert IV opioid doses to oral dosages. In either case, a bowel regimen is required to avoid potentially life-threatening constipation.

Epidural. Delivery of opioids via epidural catheter is often utilized in perioperative pain management (Breivik 2013). Together with selected local anesthetics and epinephrine, epidural opioids, especially fentanyl, contribute to "balanced analgesia" with

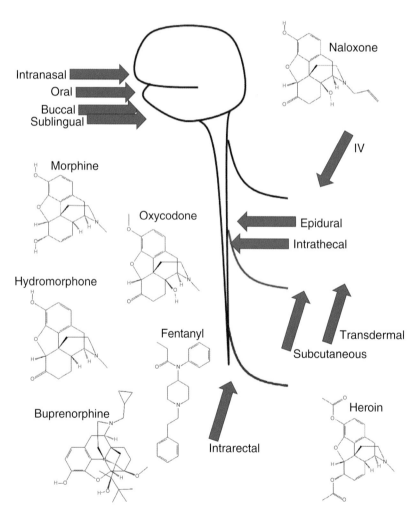

Figure 22.1 Drawing of the neuroaxis showing potential sites of opioid delivery; selected opioid and opioid antagonists are shown, see text for details.

Pain Medicine at a Glance, First Edition. Beth B. Hogans.
© 2022 John Wiley & Sons Ltd. Published 2022 by John Wiley & Sons Ltd.

multiple mechanisms of action resulting in pain control. At the same time, as reduced doses of the agents being used in combination are employed, side effects are reduced overall. Risks are discussed in more detail in Chapter 30.

Nerve blockade. Local anesthetics are used for nerve instillation in order to control pain and reduce opioid requirements perioperatively.

Transdermal. Administration of fentanyl through the skin with transdermal delivery patch application has been widely used for many years and has been tolerated in selected patients. It is important to note that **fentanyl patches should not be prescribed to opioid naïve patients**, they are only intended for patients who have already been on opioids and require round-the-clock opioid administration for pain control (Package Insert 2017). The patch should not be heated or worn during a hot bath or shower. Combination with benzodiazepines, other opioids, muscle relaxants, and drugs associated with respiratory suppression, or with alcohol can be fatal. Although a useful adjunct to therapy for patients with severe treatment resistant pain, this medication should be approached with caution as risks for substance use disorder are not insubstantial and physiological dependence will occur. As the patient typically being placed on this treatment has been treated with another opioid orally, it is important to calculate the expected morphine equivalent dosage, and then reduce the dose initially by 25–50% total to account for limited cross-tolerance upon initiation of transdermal fentanyl. For appropriate patients, limited oral rescue therapy may be provided and then the dose of transdermal fentanyl adjusted at a subsequent visit. Providers are cautioned that as with all opioids, there is physical tolerance that develops. **Dose escalation** must be approached with extreme care and avoided (Kumar et al. 2017).

Sublingual. Buprenorphine is an example of an opioid commonly delivered sublingually. Alone and in combination with naloxone, it is used in the treatment of **substance use disorder** and is **restricted** to providers that have completed advanced training and are registered to prescribe it. **Methadone** has been studied for treatment of cancer pain and in preliminary trial found safe (Hagen et al. 2010). However, there is evidence that the pain relieving effects of methadone are of shorter duration that the respiratory suppressant effects, repeated dosing of methadone to obtain pain relief can cause **toxic levels**, and potentially death, as methadone has an extremely long pharmacokinetic half-life. This approach should be limited to **specialty palliative care centers**.

Buccal. Fentanyl lozenges are available and generally only appropriate for the treatment of **advanced cancer pain**. These medications carry many **black box warnings** and even a **single lozenge may be fatal** to someone who is opioid naïve. These medications are highly subject to abuse and must be carefully secured by the patient. Providers should only prescribe this medication in a carefully defined context (Vellucci et al. 2017).

Rectal. Although rectal administration of opioids is possible, this has not gained widespread use and is currently subject to further study (Butler et al. 2017).

Subcutaneous. Administration of opioids subcutaneously is utilized in palliative care with some variation in regional practice. Nonetheless, approximately 70% of patients in palliative care will not be able to tolerate oral medication at the end of life and alternative routes are necessary (Kestenbaum et al. 2014). There is evidence to indicate that subcutaneous morphine is well tolerated and effective, the doses required may be lower than oral dosing (Masman et al. 2015).

Intranasal. Administration of naloxone intranasally is utilized in the treatment of opioid overdose. Pharmacokinetically, intranasal delivery of fentanyl results in a very rapid rise in serum levels with evident implications for potential abuse and morbidity. Nonetheless, the use of intranasal fentanyl may have a role in immediate pain control in pediatric acute care settings (Adelgais et al. 2017).

References

Adelgais, K.M., Brent, A., Wathen, J. et al. (2017). Intranasal fentanyl and quality of pediatric acute care. The Journal of Emergency Medicine 53 (5): 607–615.e2.

Breivik, H. (2013). Local anesthetic blocks and epidural analgesia. In: Chapter 37 in Wall and Melzack's Textbook of Pain, 6th Edition (eds. S. McMahon, M. Koltzenburg, I. Tracey and D. Turk).

Butler, K., Yi, J., Wasson, M. et al. (2017). Randomized controlled trial of postoperative belladonna and opium rectal suppositories in vaginal surgery. American Journal of Obstetrics and Gynecology 216 (5): 491.e1–491.e6.

Hagen, N.A., Moulin, D.E., Brasher, P.M. et al. (2010). A formal feasibility study of sublingual methadone for breakthrough cancer pain. Palliative Medicine 24 (7): 696–706.

Kestenbaum, M.G., Vilches, A.O., Messersmith, S. et al. (2014). Alternative routes to oral opioid administration in palliative care: a review and clinical summary. Pain Medicine 15 (7): 1129–1153. https://doi.org/10.1111/pme.12464. Epub 4 July 2014.

Kumar, K., Kirksey, M.A., Duong, S., and Wu, C.L. (2017). A review of opioid-sparing modalities in perioperative pain management: methods to decrease opioid use postoperatively. Anesthesia and Analgesia 125 (5): 1749–1760.

Masman, A.D., van Dijk, M., Tibboel, D. et al. (2015). Medication use during end-of-life care in a palliative care centre. International Journal of Clinical Pharmacy 37 (5): 767–775.

Janssen Pharmaceuticals. Duragesic Package Insert. Accessed April 11, 2021. https://www.accessdata.fda.gov/drugsatfda_docs/label/2005/19813s039lbl.pdf.

Vellucci, R., Mediati, R.D., Gasperoni, S. et al. (2017). Assessment and treatment of breakthrough cancer pain: from theory to clinical practice. Journal of Pain Research 10: 2147–2155. https://doi.org/10.2147/JPR.S135807. eCollection 2017.

23 Focal treatments for pain in primary practice: topical, iontophoretic, acupuncture, and basic injections

Anatomy and innervation

The focal treatment of pain is based on the idea that pain often arises from a peripheral pain generator; if it is possible to treat the pain at the source, activation of upstream pain amplification and perpetuation may be prevented. In addition, focal treatment of pain is often well received by patients who may be concerned about pills exposing the whole body to medication. Focal treatments can reduce the systemic impact and side effects of medications such as NSAIDs and steroids.

Focal treatment of pain in primary practice can involve recommending over-the-counter topical preparations, prescribing compounded neuroactive creams, providing for patients to receive iontophoretic medication, or performing basic injections within the scope of practice. Scope of practice varies with regional patterns, specialization, and advanced practice training.

Selected agents and therapies

Over the counter topicals. A range of potential therapies is available to patients as over-the-counter topical preparations, Table 23.1. These include salicylates, lidocaine, camphor and menthol, and capsaicin. Topical preparations are popular and often tried before medical care is sought for a chronic problem. The counterirritants, e.g. **camphor** and **menthol**, are especially helpful for musculoskeletal pain. **Salicylate** containing preparations may be useful for acute arthritis flares however use may lead to systemic levels. **Capsaicin** containing creams temporarily disrupt the distal nerve endings and produce strong burning sensations. Capsaicin creams must be applied 4–5 times daily with gloves; contact with mucous membranes (eyes) is distinctly painful. Joints that are close to the surface, e.g. knees and shoulders, respond better to capsaicin than deeper joints like hip and spine; **patients with neuropathy should avoid capsaicin** as increased pain may result. **Lidocaine** may be effective in nociceptive, inflammatory, and neuropathic pain, safety concerns limit amounts used.

Prescription topicals. A few medications are available for use as prescription topicals. Voltaren gel contains ketorolac and is applied up to four times daily. An NSAID, this is most useful for additional relief of single arthritic joint pain.

Compounded preparations. Compounded medicines got a bad reputation in the 2011 when patients were sickened by tainted steroid solutions. In that case, preservative-free steroid solution was prepared under improper conditions leading to severe fungal infections when injected. Compounded preparations do not have FDA approval in most cases but RCTs are accruing, Table 23.2, (Cline and Turrentine 2016). Gabapentin, Ketamine, Baclofen, Amitriptyline, and Ibuprofen can be compounded together or separately to make a topical. For some patients this approach reduces side effects from systemic administration.

Iontophoresis. Some medications can be delivered through the skin with electrical current. Utilized in physical therapy, this can deliver steroids to specific areas, such as lateral epicondyle. This application is distinct from the use of iontophoretic patches to deliver medications systemically.

Table 23.1 Over-the-counter topical agents and preparations.

Compound	Strength (examples)	Trade name (examples)	Intended use	Frequency of dosing	Notes
Menthol	4, 10%	Biofreeze	Aches, pains, strains and sprains	Every six hours as needed, no more than three times daily	Do not occlude, heat, or apply to broken skin or mucous membranes
Trolamine salicylate 10%	10%	Aspercreme	Arthritis, muscle aches	No more than four times daily	Do not occlude, heat or apply to broken skin or mucous membranes
Lidocaine	4%	Icy Hot, Gold Bond, Salon Pas, Aspercreme with lidocaine	Numbing	Every six hours as needed, no more than three times daily	Do not occlude, heat or apply to a large area
Methylsalicylate	30% in combination with other agents	BenGay	Aches, pains, strains and sprains	Every six hours as needed, no more than three times daily	Do not occlude, heat or apply to broken skin or mucous membranes
Camphor	11%	Combined with menthol in Tiger Balm	Aches, pains, strains and sprains	Every six hours as needed, no more than three times daily	Do not occlude, heat or apply to broken skin or mucous membranes
Capsaicin	0.0025%	Capsaicin	Aches, pains	five times daily	Makes neuropathy pain worse in many

Allergic reactions are a contraindication to treatment with topical agents.

Pain Medicine at a Glance, First Edition. Beth B. Hogans.
© 2022 John Wiley & Sons Ltd. Published 2022 by John Wiley & Sons Ltd.

Table 23.2 Prescription topical agents.

Compound	Strength (examples)	Intended use	Notes
Diclofenac (Voltaren gel)	1, 3%	Arthritis pain	Dose limited, twice daily
Gabapentin	2–6%	Vulvodynia	RCT in 2008 for vulvodynia
Clonidine	0.2%	Neuralgia, orofacial pain	Multiple RCTs show efficacy, side effects limit use
Amitriptyline	4%	Chemotherapy & PHN	Compounded with baclofen and ketamine RCT shows efficacy
Baclofen	2%	—	—
Ketamine	1, 2%	—	—

PHN post-herpetic neuralgia, *RCT* randomized controlled trial.

Acupuncture. Acupuncture has been shown effective in selected conditions with RCT and high level evidence. Acupuncture training currently requires 300 hours of coursework and additional time to acquire clinical expertise. It is a useful complement to some pain treatment plans although in many cases a series of treatments, e.g., 10–12, is necessary to attain a benefit, and insurance coverage may be limited or non-existent. Many patients are quite interested in a trial of acupuncture.

Trigger point injections. Barbara Travell, White House physician during the Kennedy and Johnson administrations popularized the use of trigger point injections for the relief of chronic pain. Presented in authoritative detail in a two-volume text co-authored with David Simon, Travell set forth an enduring foundation for clinical assessment and treatment of trigger point related pain conditions (Travell and Simons 1998). Trigger points have been studied by Jay Shah and colleagues who demonstrated **high levels of inflammatory mediators present in active trigger points** (Shah et al. 2008). These taut bands and areas of focal muscle contraction can be treated through massage, self-massage, injections of saline, lidocaine, or "dry-needling" (Davies 2013).

Botox injections. Botulinum toxin is used to paralyze muscles and may be useful in the relief of chronic pain associated with muscle spasm and with headache. There has been use in chronic neuropathic pain but this is a specialist application. Botox remains expensive, but for some patients it is a useful adjunct with relatively few problematic side effects. Training workshops are available to prepare the interested provider in this technique.

Basic nerve blocks. Basic nerve blocks, particularly the greater occipital nerve block, can be performed in primary care and specialty care settings with sufficient training and experience. There is some evidence to indicate that this may be a useful complement in managing cervicogenic headache (Kleen and Levin 2016).

Intraarticular injections of steroid. Selected joint injections can be performed in **primary care and specialty care** settings providing that the clinician has had adequate training in **protocols, procedures, safety, and failure modes**. There is an increasing trend to utilize **ultrasound** for localization; to avoid injection of blood vessels and nerves. Efficacy varies with site: there is evidence to indicate that steroid injections for adhesive capsulitis of the shoulder can provide early pain relief, but outcomes are unchanged a one-year timepoints (Ranalletta et al. 2016). There evidence for intra-articular steroids to the knee is more mixed (Jüni et al. 2015). One study suggests that warfarin treatment may not be a contraindication to joint injection treatment (Bashir et al. 2015).

Although steroids are often delivered focally for the treatment of pain, **systemic steroids** should be approached with **caution** (Madalena and Lerch 2017). Short courses of steroids, e.g. pulse-taper, are often used for acute nerve compression or spondylosis-related pain flairs. Longer-term use of steroids is associated with more harms than benefits and should be limited to specific rheumatological conditions (Strehl et al. 2016).

References

Bashir, M.A., Ray, R., Sarda, P. et al. (2015). Determination of a safe INR for joint injections in patients taking warfarin. Annals of the Royal College of Surgeons of England 97 (8): 589–591.

Cline, A.E. and Turrentine, J.E. (2016). Compounded topical analgesics for chronic pain. Dermatitis 27 (5): 263–271.

Davies, C. (2013). Trigger Point Therapy Workbook. New Harbinger Press.

Jüni, P., Hari, R., Rutjes, A.W. et al. (2015). Intra-articular corticosteroid for knee osteoarthritis. Cochrane Database of Systematic Reviews 10: CD005328.

Kleen, J.K. and Levin, M. (2016). Injection therapy for headache and facial pain. Oral and Maxillofacial Surgery Clinics of North America 28 (3): 423–434.

Madalena, K.M. and Lerch, J.K. (2017). The effect of glucocorticoid and glucocorticoid receptor interactions on brain, spinal cord, and glial cell plasticity. Neural Plasticity 2017: 8640970.

Ranalletta, M., Rossi, L.A., Bongiovanni, S.L. et al. (2016). Corticosteroid injections accelerate pain relief and recovery of function compared with oral NSAIDs in patients with adhesive capsulitis: a randomized controlled trial. The American Journal of Sports Medicine 44 (2): 474–481.

Shah, J.P., Danoff, J.V., Desai, M.J. et al. (2008). Biochemicals associated with pain and inflammation are elevated in sites near to and remote from active myofascial trigger points. Archives of Physical Medicine and Rehabilitation 89 (1): 16–23.

Strehl, C., Bijlsma, J.W., de Wit, M. et al. (2016). Defining conditions where long-term glucocorticoid treatment has an acceptably low level of harm to facilitate implementation of existing recommendations: viewpoints from an EULAR task force. Annals of the Rheumatic Diseases 75 (6): 952–957. https://doi.org/10.1136/annrheumdis-2015-208916. Epub 2016 Mar 1.

Travell, B. and Simons, D. (1998). Myofascial Pain and Dysfunction: The Trigger Point Manual, 2nde, vol. 2. LWW.

Interventional pain management techniques may provide urgently needed pain relief but should occur **within the context of a comprehensive approach to pain**. Several interventional approaches provide temporary pain relief; physical activity and therapy are needed for functional restoration so that when the pain injection wears off, the patient will be better than before. Pain injections almost always contain steroids and have infection risks. Systemic steroid effects, such as diabetes and osteoporosis, limit re-injections. There are risks for local damage as the needle enters the body and approaches close to the nerve. Nerve damage can induce persistent pain. For these reasons, technical expertise is essential.

Surgical approaches impacting pain care are two principle types: surgery intended to impact the pain-processing system itself, and surgery intended to correct a problem leading to persistent activation of peripheral pain generators, e.g. joint replacement surgery.

LESI or Lumbar epidural steroid injection involves injection of **local anesthetic and steroid near a lumbar nerve root** (Figure 24.1). The local anesthetic temporarily numbs the nerve but wears off within hours. The steroid component, usually a **long-acting steroid**, is not immediately effective so that the patient may experience temporary **re-emergence of pain** the night of the injection followed by gradual **relief of pain** that may persist for some weeks. Some specialists also include a shorter-acting steroid in the injectate. The safety of LESI performed by experienced practitioners is well-established but there are limitations, including HPA suppression (Abdul et al. 2017). The American Academy of Neurology discourages use of LESI despite the evidence for **effective pain relief over the 2 to 6-week time frame** citing lack of efficacy at 24 hours and 1-year (AAN Summary of Evidence-based Guideline for CLINICIANS 2017). For some patients' pain relief over the intermediate timeframe is useful to complement oral analgesia and allow rehabilitational therapies.

CESI. Cervical epidural steroid injection is less widely practiced due to relatively more challenging anatomy. Short, horizontally-oriented nerve roots mean the spinal cord is near the treatment needle. Performance by a practitioner highly experienced in this technique is essential.

Nerve ablation. As a hypothetical, it might seem expedient to eliminate a pain problem by cutting or destroying the nerve to a painful structure. Practical experience has demonstrated that nerves often grow back and patients have insidious and troublesome **recurrence of pain after a period** of relief lasting days to weeks. Patients can develop severe, treatment resistant **denervation pain** (anesthesia dolorosa). Nerve ablation can be done using a variety of techniques in carefully selected patients, and may be useful in managing severe pain for patients with **limited life expectancy**.

Spinal cord stimulation. Implantation of specialized **electrodes over the dorsal column of the spinal cord** has been developed as a technique for the treatment of severe, treatment-resistant pain (Figure 24.2). Utilized for forms of pain such as Chronic Regional Pain Syndrome, atypical somatic, and chronic limb pain, the treatment is effective in carefully selected patients. The pain is replaced in most cases by a **tingling sensation** (paresthesia). Medication is still needed in most but at **reduced doses**, potentially with less severe side effects. As with all implantable devices there is the risk of infection which can necessitate removal of the device.

Indwelling pump. In some patients, placement of a permanent or indwelling catheter supplying medication to the **epidural** or **intrathecal** space is a useful treatment option (Figure 24.3). In the ideal scenario, indwelling catheter delivery systems allow for **targeted drug delivery** and avoidance of **systemic side effects** which can be profoundly impairing. As with spinal cord stimulators, there are risks associated with implantable devices. In addition, there are risks associated with sudden medication stoppage due to catheter blockage or reservoir problems, and risks associated with medication overdose if an error occurs during the **refilling procedure**.

Joint replacement surgery. Replacement of knee and hip joints is very common in the United States, millions of Americans live with these devices (Kremers et al. 2014). This is an important form of pain management intervention as the vast majority of procedures are performed to address painful dysfunction of a joint due to advanced arthritis not amenable to other treatments (Wolford et al. 2015). In the field of joint replacement, it is clear that **reliably**

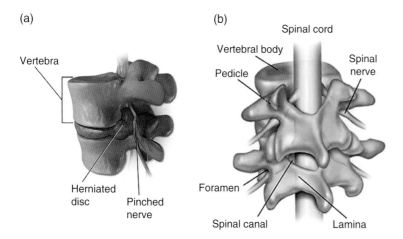

(a)

Vertebra

Herniated disc

Pinched nerve

(b)

Spinal cord

Vertebral body

Pedicle

Spinal nerve

Foramen

Spinal canal

Lamina

Figure 24.1 Spinal column views with (a) herniated disc compressing nerve root, and (b) normal appearance showing anatomical relationships.

Pain Medicine at a Glance, First Edition. Beth B. Hogans.
© 2022 John Wiley & Sons Ltd. Published 2022 by John Wiley & Sons Ltd.

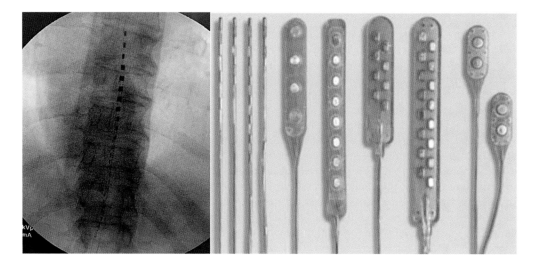

Figure 24.2 Spinal cord stimulator illustration. Source: North, R. B. et al. (2019) and Epstein, L. J., & Palmieri, M. (2012). © John Wiley & Sons.

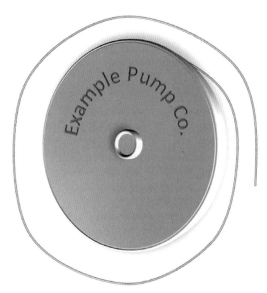

Figure 24.3 Spinal cord indwelling pump illustration.

excellent perioperative pain control is essential to promoting better clinical outcomes, reducing complications, and advancing the pace of rehabilitation, see Chapter 30.

Spinal surgery. The spine is subject to several forms of damage or degeneration amenable to surgical management. Procedures include: microdiscectomy, laminectomy, single-level fusion, and heavily instrumented multilevel fusion. Artificial discs can be placed, and rods, plates, and screws can be used to **stabilize structures** and **alleviate pressure** on vital nerve structures. Patient selection is very important including both **psychological appropriateness** and **medical comorbidities**. The risks for muscle deconditioning are serious and should be addressed preoperatively whenever possible with PT consultation in advance of surgery. Advances in perioperative pain control have improved the course and outcome of rehabilitation after surgery.

Neurosurgery. There is an established history of neurosurgical procedures targeting disruption of CNS pain processing. Although each procedure has particular success rates and associated risks, procedures such as cutting of the dorsal root, removal of the dorsal root ganglion, and sectioning of the spinal cord in posterior columns and the anterior midline, are associated with early initial pain relief followed by gradual increases in patients experiencing pain such that outcomes at one year post-operative are overall unfavorable (Dorsi and Lenz 2013). Careful consideration of risks and benefits must be weighed before proceeding. More recently, **implantable stimulation techniques**, e.g. cortical stimulation, and deep brain stimulation, show some promise (Linderoth and Meyerson 2013).

References

AAN Summary of Evidence-based Guideline for CLINICIANS (2017). Use of epidural steroid injections to treat radicular lumbosacral pain. Minneapolis, MN. https://www.aan.com/Guidelines/Home/GetGuidelineContent/250 (accessed 13 December 2017).

Abdul, A.J., Ghai, B., Bansal, D. et al. (2017). Hypothalamic pituitary adrenocortical axis suppression following a single epidural injection of methylprednisolone acetate. Pain Physician 20 (7): E991–E1001.

Dorsi, M. and Lenz, F. (2013). *Neurosurgical Approaches to the Treatment of Pain. Chapter 40 in Wall and Melzack's Textbook of Pain*, 6the (eds. S. McMahon, M. Koltzenburg, I. Tracey and D. Turk).

Linderoth, B. and Meyerson, B. (2013). *Spinal Cord and Brain Stimulation. Chapter 41 in Wall and Melzack's Textbook of Pain*, 6the (eds. S. Mcmahon, M. Koltzenburg, I. Tracey and D. Turk).

Kremers HM, et al. (2014). Prevalence of total hip (THA) and total knee (TKA) arthroplasty in the United States. Presentation at: *American Academy of Orthopaedic Surgeons Annual Meeting*, 2014, New Orleans, La.

Wolford, M.L., Palso, K., and Bercovitz, A. (2015). Hospitalization for total hip replacement among inpatients aged 45 and over: United States, 2000–2010. NCHS Data Brief No. 186.

The importance of engaging patients in activating treatments for persistent pain cannot be overstated. Cognitive therapies, discussed in the next chapter, include awakening patient's awareness to the capacity to change their fate: appropriate utilization of activating therapies is the most critical element within a patient's control (Figure 25.1). As providers, it is essential that we effectively communicate about activating therapies and our confidence that these therapies, correctly applied, are highly effective (Table 25.1). **Unless a patient engages in some form of activating therapy, the chance of resolving a chronic pain problem is slim.** Relying entirely on passive strategies such as injections, surgeries, and even pill-taking leads to a state of worsening pain and potentially life-threatening complications. Like a spotlight, we can highlight the best choices for our patients, and like a coach move them to get engaged. There are many forms of activating therapies, it is important to discover, through **values-based conversation**, which of these therapies is most aligned with the patient's health-related values (Figure 25.2). Then make specific shared-decision-making plans for treatment. If basic guidance does not prompt positive behavior change, e.g. engaging in a 20-minute daily walk, then with motivational interviewing,

Daily stretching   Tailored exercise   Core

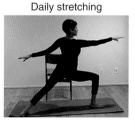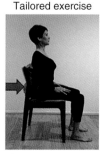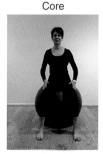

Figure 25.2 Examples of activating therapies.

we identify with the patient goals that are **"SMART" goals: specific, measurable, attainable, relevant, and time-bound**. Clinical psychology research shows these are more effective in motivating positive change.

Physical/occupational therapy. Physical therapy is the foundation of **opioid-sparing treatment** of most pain-associated conditions. PT can be useful both before and after joint replacement. Obviously, PT is essential for rehabilitation of sprains and strains, but **also for neuropathic pain conditions** where challenges of balance and gait can predominate. Depending on the pain-associated condition at hand, you may need PT providers who are especially attuned to relevant concerns. Get to know your local physical therapy practitioners and ask your patients for feedback about their experiences. When writing a PT prescription: (i) provide your working diagnosis, (ii) specify evaluation and management, and (iii) request a report so that you can review the appraisal. Often the physical therapist has valuable insight and identifies associated problems such as **postural flaws** or another diagnosis causing pain perpetuation. Good PT must lead to a realistic home exercise program to solidifying therapy gains.

Exercise. It is essential that patients identify an appealing exercise regimen and vital that providers ask patients about exercise activities. Both **cardio and strength training** have beneficial effects in most pain-associated conditions. Cardio intensity depends on cardiac and neurologic fitness however, moderate daily exercise such as 20–30 minutes of walking is a baseline level for most older adults. Higher levels of intensity such as jogging, running, or swimming are beneficial for most young and middle-aged adults. Strength training has been demonstrated as effective in decreasing chronic pain. **Older patients** also benefit. Provide specific detail about performing strength training at least three times weekly, and follow up.

Hydrotherapy. Water buoyancy can mitigate instability, unload painful joints from gravitational stress, provide relaxation, and facilitate strengthening and stretching. Patients often respond to hydrotherapy as a safe and supportive environment to overcome otherwise overwhelming pain with movement. Importantly,

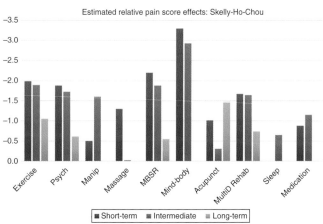

Estimated relative pain score effects: Skelly-Ho-Chou

Figure 25.1 Estimated relative pain Score impacts for chronic pain.

Table 25.1 Activating therapies, evidence base and applications.

Therapy	Evidence	Applications
Physical therapy	Extremely Strong	Multiple conditions
Moderate daily exercise	Strong	FM, chronic pain
Strength training	Good	Chronic pain
Yoga	Strong	Chronic pain
Chi gong	Emerging	Chronic pain
Sleep	Good	Chronic pain

Pain Medicine at a Glance, First Edition. Beth B. Hogans.
© 2022 John Wiley & Sons Ltd. Published 2022 by John Wiley & Sons Ltd.

patients with **arthritis will need a warm pool** environment whereas patients with underlying **neuropathic conditions require cool water**, e.g., MS deficits worsen dramatically with elevated core temperature.

Yoga and chi gong. Eastern approaches to health, movement, flexibility, and balance have gained widespread acceptance. The benefits of Yoga are well known and forms of yoga are multiple (Groess et al. 2017). If a person is not versed in yoga, a gentle beginning is preferable. Some patients, especially "Type A" personalities, will overdo yoga, potentially creating more problems. Encourage patients to learn about **internal yoga processes** to modulate the physical efforts being made (Boccio and Feuerstein 1993; NurrieStearns 2010). One example is over-flexing the spine in a cat-cow dynamic pose. Excessive arching in the "cat" position can worsen thoracic kyphosis pain. Check in with the patient doing yoga and have them demonstrate some poses. Chi gong (Qi gong) or Tai Chi is a form of **moving meditation**. Ideal for balance, feelings of centeredness, increased energy and stress relief, there are multiple resources available and emerging evidence of efficacy against pain (Bai et al. 2015). Sometimes available as an open-air practice, there are also excellent video programs to teach this practice in private (Holden 2017).

Sleep. Perhaps it's ironic to call sleep an activating treatment, however improving sleep is a study in managing behaviors and taking active steps toward change. A strong commitment is essential to success. Sleep, like exercise, has protean effects on pain processing. There is a reciprocal relationship in which poor sleep leads to worsening pain, and worsened pain leads to poorer sleep. Although there are many medications sold for sleep, it is essential to work on **sleep hygiene** as part of any program to improve sleep. Begin by asking patients about their sleep, Table 25.2. A brief list of sleep hygiene tips should be discussed with the patient and handouts provided, e.g. Sleep countdown (Table 25.3). It is important to check back with patients about their sleep at each visit in which pain is discussed. Formal scales are available to measure sleep quality (Broderick et al. 2013), referral to a sleep specialist may be necessary and appraisal of possible sleep apnea may be appropriate in patients with obesity, hypertension, reflux, and daytime sleepiness. **Obstructive sleep apnea** is present in 25% of older adult males and 10% of older adult females.

Table 25.2 Common sleep questions.

What time do you get into bed?
What time do you get out of bed?
How long are your awake before falling asleep?
What time do you wake up?
How often do you wake up early?
How many times at night do you wake up?
Do you have a T.V. in your bedroom?
How much does pain interfere with your sleep?

Table 25.3 Daily sleep countdown.

Countdown time	Activity
T – 6 h	No more caffeine or chocolate
T – 90 min	Stop TV/computer/phone/ screen watching
T – 60 min	Have a light snack and relax
T – 45 min	Dim the lights
T – 30 min	Have a comforting bedtime ritual, e.g. bathing, calming music, guided imagery
T = Bedtime	Calculate how many hours you sleep. Subtract back from when you need to get up and go to bed at that time
T + 7–8 h	Get out of bed when the alarm first goes off
T + 8 h	Sleep in no more than one extra hour on days off

It is associated with less sleep, lower sleep quality, cognitive impairments, CAD and stroke (Olaithe et al. 2017). Shortened sleep duration increases persistent pain (Mundt et al. 2017). Screening and referral are essential.

References

Bai, Z., Guan, Z., Fan, Y. et al. (2015). The effects of qigong for adults with chronic pain: systematic review and meta-analysis. The American Journal of Chinese Medicine 43 (8): 1525–1539.

Boccio, F.J. and Feuerstein, G. (1993). Mindfulness Yoga: The Awakened Union of Breath, Body, and Mind. Wisdom Publications 9 January 1993.

Broderick, J.E., Junghaenel, D.U., Schneider, S. et al. (2013). Pittsburgh and Epworth sleep scale items: accuracy of ratings across different reporting periods. Behavioral Sleep Medicine 11: 173–188.

Groess, E.J., Liu, L., Chang, D.G. et al. (2017). Yoga for military veterans with chronic low back pain: a randomized clinical trial. The American Journal of Preventive Medicine 53 (5): 599–608.

Holden, L. (2017). Qi Gong Flow for Beginners, DVD. http://www.exercisetoheal.com/Qi+Gong+DVDs/Qi+Gong+Flow+for+Beginners.html (accessed 13 December 2017).

Mundt, J.M., Eisenschenk, S., and Robinson, M.E. (2017). An examination of pain's relationship to sleep fragmentation and disordered breathing across common sleep disorders. Pain Medicine https://doi.org/10.1093/pm/pnx211. [Epub ahead of print].

NurrieStearns, M. (2010). Yoga for Anxiety: Meditations and Practices for Calming the Body and Mind. New Harbinger Publications 2 February 2010.

Olaithe, M., Bucks, R.S., Hillman, D.R., and Eastwood, P.R. (2018). Cognitive deficits in obstructive sleep apnea: Insights from a meta-review and comparison with deficits observed in COPD, insomnia, and sleep deprivation. Sleep Medicine Reviews 38: 39–49. pii: S1087-0792(17)30070-9.

The brain is both the seat of pain perception and the repository of our most powerful personal tools against pain: we can engage in healthier lifestyles, and we can change how we think and feel. In **Cognitive Behavioral Therapy** (CBT), people learn to think about themselves differently and pursue better choices; Learning how situational triggers, automatic erroneous thoughts, reactive feelings, and undesirable behaviors contribute to persistent pain. In **Acceptance Commitment Therapy** (ACT), people learn to pull back from their thought-dominated experience of life and enmeshment with emotions; and then direct their energies more fully into meaningful activities. New treatment modes are in development, including "Emotional awareness and expression therapy" (Bellomo et al. 2020). Much has been learned about the brain and pain in the last 40 years. By integrating some basic clinical psychology into clinical practice, it is possible to take the first steps in helping people **live better despite** their **pain**. In addition, by welcoming clinical psychology methods with **intentionality**, we ease the transition for our patients who ultimately pursue full clinical psychology.

At present, there are not enough clinical psychologists trained in pain to meet the needs. Beyond this, many insurance companies will not pay for these treatments; It takes a highly motivated patient, willing to pay out-of-pocket, to seek out an experienced provider and take the time to learn these methods. Therefore, it is vital that primary care providers learn to implement clinical psychological approaches to pain management in everyday practice, even if an **eclectic** approach is utilized (Altman 2014).

The first step is to put the patient at the center. Then it is essential to guide the patient in understanding that they have some **power over pain**. You can learn more here, in Appendix 5, and from the references for this chapter.

CBT: CBT posits that we respond to adverse events with erroneous thoughts, alarming emotions, and untoward behaviors, Figure 26.1. In cognitive behavior therapy, multiple therapeutic steps are taken in sequence (Otis 2007; Darnall 2016), Table 26.1. At the core of CBT is **relaxation** (Lebovits 2007). **Gaining control over the level of arousal** is critically important to the subsequent steps because a person who is in a chronic state of heightened arousal cannot absorb and consistently apply productive changes (Herman 2015). Relaxation can include **diaphragmatic breathing**, guided imagery, meditation, **biofeedback**, or hypnosis. Next is **cognitive restructuring**. In this phase of CBT, patients learn to recognize automatic thoughts, cognitive errors associated with these thoughts, Table 26.2, links between stressful experiences and automatic thoughts, and begin to re-appraise automatic thoughts and replace them with more reflective appraisals. **Stress management** is an active multidimensional aspect of CBT that includes **recognizing triggers, containing stressful events, pacing, scheduling pleasant activities, managing anger**, and **improving sleep**. The final stage is to put the parts together so that there is **always a plan** to handle **pain emergencies**. Barriers to CBT include time and money costs, lack of primary care buy

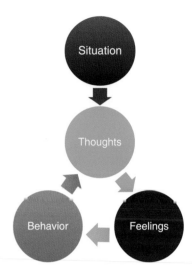

Figure 26.1 CBT: a situation leads to thoughts which produce feelings that lead to behaviors. This is also presented as the a-b-c model where (a) is for activating event, (b) is for beliefs (misbeliefs) and (c) is for consequences, e.g. feelings and reactions ensuing from the event.

Table 26.1 Elements of cognitive behavioral therapy.

Relaxation	Cognitive restructuring	Stress management
Recognizing the links between tension and pain	Recognizing the leaps from events to thoughts	Recognizing the stress response as it occurs
Diaphragmatic breathing	Learning about automatic thoughts	Time-based pacing
Guided imagery	Recognizing types of cognitive errors	Scheduled pleasant activities
Hypnosis	Replacing errors with positive appraisals	Sleep: conditioned responses
Progressive muscle relaxation	Keeping track of thoughts and appraisals	Managing anger by responding assertively
Meditation	Reflecting on progress	Planning for emergencies

in, weak patient commitment, and technical inconsistencies. Nonetheless, there is good evidence that CBT is **safe and effective** for chronic pain. Each CBT element may be useful to patients and can be introduced in a primary care setting (Otis 2007); however, the evidence base for CBT as effective is primarily based on coordinated implementation.

ACT: In Acceptance Commitment Therapy, the patient **recommits to life** dedicated to their dearest values (Oliver et al. 2016). ACT arises from Western adaptations of Eastern philosophy (Hayes and Smith 2005). This is the origin of the term "acceptance" which can have a **negative connotation** for many patients who surmise that acceptance means accepting limitations imposed on them externally. Nonetheless, the core idea is that **we do not consist of our thoughts, our feelings, or even the sum of our suffering**. We have the capacity

Pain Medicine at a Glance, First Edition. Beth B. Hogans.
© 2022 John Wiley & Sons Ltd. Published 2022 by John Wiley & Sons Ltd.

Table 26.2 Errors of thought contributing to pain perpetuation.

Intensive negative focus
Discounting the positive
All-or-none thinking
Leaping to conclusions
Overgeneralization
Catastrophizing
Rumination
Pejorative self-labeling
Self-referential thoughts
Identification with feelings
False obligations ("shoulds")

Table 26.3 Six elements of acceptance-commitment therapy.

Experiential avoidance: acting to avoid feeling bad
Fusion: not separating the self from thoughts
Inflexibility: adhering to an unproductive narrative of self
Losing contact with the present moment
Not connecting with deepest values
Failure of committed action

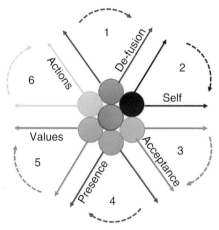

Figure 26.2 The six "pivots" of ACT, adapted from Stephen Hayes. In ACT, the patient pivots from focus on the external world to the "self", from a state of fusion with events to constructive "de-fusion", from operating consistent with expectations to discovering "values", from a state of struggle to "acceptance", and from inaction, to a life of "actions" that express "values" and raise awareness of self in relation to defuse reality.

to separate a part of ourselves, often referred to the as "the **core self**" or simply "the self" and hold that self apart from the mental chatter and waves of emotion (Figure 26.2). In doing this, it is possible to rededicate energy and attention towards those things that bring us joy and meaning, Table 26.3. ACT has been extensively studied and is an evidenced-based practice for the treatment of chronic pain.

If you can refer someone to a pain-specializing clinical psychologist, the referral typically requires preparation in order to have the patient embrace referral and follow through successfully. We are not referring them to psychology because they are hopeless or because the problem is in their head, but rather because they have options. This **is one option that is particularly free from bothersome side effects** (ideal for people who don't like to rely on medications), and the *solution* to their pain is potentially in their head, or *more precisely by changing their thoughts, feelings, and behaviors.* The psychologist can teach them to **utilize their natural strengths more effectively**. Building an alliance and letting the patient know that referral to psychology does not mean the end of your established therapeutic relationship is valuable, assure the patient that you will

continue to meet with them while they are seeing the psychologist and that your treatments will complement those of the psychologist. Especially if you have already implemented some of the methods of clinical psychology in your work with the patient, you can point to these aspects of the treatment and highlight how this is one part of what the psychologist would work with them on, and that a fuller implementation of psychological therapies will be even more helpful. Profound insights into one's personal power and liberation from the bonds of pain await the patient who is willing to try this avenue of treatment (Miller and Jenkins 2006).

References

Altman, D. (2014). The Mindfulness Toolbox, 50 practical tips, tools, and handouts for anxiety, depression, and pain. Eau Claire, Wisconsin: PESI Publishing and Media.

Bellomo, T.R., Schrepf, A., Kruger, G.H. et al. (2020). Pressure pain tolerance predicts the success of emotional awareness and expression therapy in patients with fibromyalgia. The Clinical Journal of Pain 36 (7): 562–566.

Darnall, B. (2016). Opioid-Free Pain Relief Kit: 10 Simple Steps to Ease Your Pain Kindle, 1e. Bull Publishing Company 1 July 2016.

Herman, J.L. (2015). Trauma and Recovery: The Aftermath of Violence--From Domestic Abuse to Political Terror, 1Re. Basic Books 7 July 2015.

Lebovits, A. (2007). Cognitive-behavioral approaches to chronic pain. Primary Psychiatry 14 (9): 2007. http://primarypsychiatry.com/cognitive-behavioral-approaches-to-chronic-pain/ (accessed 8 December 2017).

Miller, A. and Jenkins, A. (2006). The Body Never Lies: The Lingering Effects of Hurtful Parenting. W. W. Norton & Company Reprint edition. 17 August 2006.

Oliver, J., Hill, J., and Morris, E. (2016). ACTivate Your Life: Using Acceptance and Mindfulness to Build a Life That is Rich, Fulfilling and Fun Paperback. Constable and Robinson Publishers 2 August 2016.

Otis, J. (2007). Managing Chronic Pain: A Cognitive-Behavioral Therapy Approach Workbook (Treatments That Work) Workbook Edition. Oxford University Press Workbook edition. 24 September 2007.

Hayes, S.C. and Smith, S. (2005). Get Out of Your Mind and Into Your Life: The New Acceptance and Commitment Therapy (A New Harbinger Self-Help Workbook) Paperback. Oakland, CA: New Harbinger Publications 1 November 2005.

Manual therapies including massage, trigger point therapies, acupressure, chiropractic, stretching, traction, and inversion are among the most effective and safest therapies available for musculoskeletal conditions. Although musculoskeletal conditions are the most common cause of pain globally, many people don't have reliable access to these important treatment modalities. Insurance may not include these therapies except as part of PT or chiropractic treatment. Healthcare providers need to know these therapies and recommend them appropriately. Especially trigger points are under-appreciated and can hugely impact quality of life through self-management.

Massage therapy has multiple different forms of varying efficacy. Although widely held not to be effective for the long-term pain reduction, there is evidence of substantive short-term relief (Davies and Davies 2013). Massage therapy that targets deep tissue, myofascial tissue, or trigger points can play an important role in rapidly correcting maladaptive movement patterns and offering patients the instant relief that make pills and injections so appealing. It is useful to know of qualified practitioners in your area to provide referrals for patients. Two modalities will be discussed in detail here: trigger point and acupressure massage; although both involve focal pressure, the former arises from myofascial approaches while the latter developed from acupuncture. Massaging pillows, pads, and handheld devices may be a cost-effective way for patients who cannot afford the high out-of-pocket costs of individualized massage therapy, to attain some relief.

Trigger points are palpable firm "knots" present in large and small muscle groups (Simons et al. 1999). Trigger points are termed "active" if pain is present and "latent" if not. It is important to palpate with the pads of the fingers using moderate pressure with circular motion to assess for these. Trapezius trigger points are nearly universally present in adult females and very prevalent in males (Figure 27.1). These muscle abnormalities were described in detail by Janet Travell, who with David Simons coauthored the definitive scholarly work. She identified predictable patterns of referred pain arising from trigger points, relieved by treatment. A useful practical manual, highly recommended for all healthcare providers interested in pain, authored by Claire and Amber Davies, is now in third edition. Once viewed with skepticism by academics; trigger points were studied by Jay Shah and colleagues at the NIH who used microcatheters to measure inflammatory mediators including NGF, TNF-alpha, and norepinephrine (Shah et al. 2008). Patients can learn to identify and self-manage trigger points, potentially important for cervicogenic headache and postural back pain. Treatment of trigger points may help restore blood flow and facilitate muscle repair. Passive approaches to trigger point treatment exist but some result in healthcare "churning".

Acupressure massage is based on Chinese medicine and uses pressure at specific sites. Acupressure may relieve migraine, stress, anxiety, insomnia, and other symptoms contributing to pain and suffering. Intriguingly, the acupressure points for relief of migraine

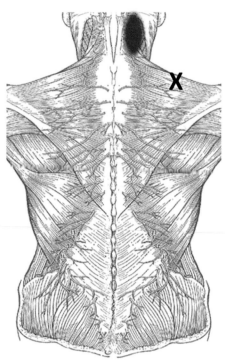

Figure 27.1 Massage therapy – trigger points, X indicates location of trigger point site in muscle, red-shared area indicates location of referred pain.

are near Botox injection points, suggesting a convergence of mechanisms (Figure 27.2). Michael Gach has written a useful reference manual (Gach 2011). Patients may be very interested in this therapy; provider engagement around this alternative approach can strengthen rapport and enhance a patient's receptiveness to other therapies and pain-relieving lifestyle changes.

Chiropractic therapy can enhance management of many forms of musculoskeletal pain. Chiropractors are trained in manual therapy and chiropractic adjustment. Foundational education lasts about three years and focuses on spinal and para-spinal realignment techniques. Although there have been occasional reports of stroke associated with high velocity cervical (neck) adjustments, modern chiropractic methods are very safe and typically provide immediate relief. It may be important to couple chiropractic with physical therapy-based exercise in order attain sustained results, i.e. correct maladaptive movement patterns, to free patients from dependence on repeated chiropractic adjustments.

Stretching improves musculoskeletal health and function. If you maintain a seated position while working, the hip flexors progressively shorten, ultimately impeding people from standing fully erect. This flexed hip posture increases lumbar hyperlordosis and cervical extension. Next time you are people-watching – look to see how many older adults walk with a stooped forward posture – this

Pain Medicine at a Glance, First Edition. Beth B. Hogans.
© 2022 John Wiley & Sons Ltd. Published 2022 by John Wiley & Sons Ltd.

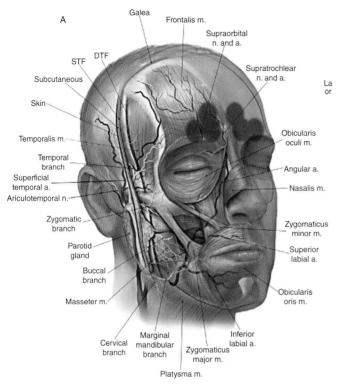

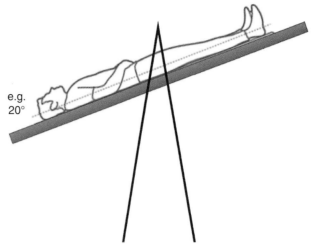

Figure 27.4 Inversion table illustration, please observe appropriate clinical precautions in use.

Figure 27.2 Example of acupressure points in forehead. Source: Christensen et al (2015). © John Wiley & Sons.

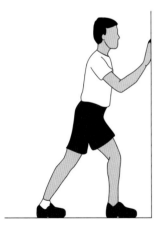

Figure 27.3 Lunge stretch illustration, stretching routines should be personalized to patient, their physical capacities, and pain needs. Source: Foot and Ankle Conditioning Program. Reproduced with permission from OrthoInfo. © American Academy of Orthopaedic Surgeons. https://orthoinfo.org/

may not be a consequence of back pain – it may be a contributor! A gentle forward lunge with conscious hip extension twice a day may be enough to prevent chronic hip flexor contracture (Figure 27.3). Stretching is important for the prevention and management of many chronic musculoskeletal pains, please see the Appendix for a handy guide to daily stretches for healthy movement.

Traction can be an important component of manual therapy depending on the circumstance. Although some studies have suggested traction is not effective for LBP, due to our upright posture and the effects of gravity, it may be that traction can help alleviate chronic pain and restore blood flow to promote healing. Manual leg traction can be helpful in alleviative musculoskeletal hip pain due to muscle spasm or misalignment. Certainly, when muscle contracture is present, traction may be indicated and can help patients.

Inversion or positional therapy can be useful in some patients but must be used with caution. Although large studies have not been performed, it is prudent to refrain from inversion in the elderly, patients with high blood pressure or a personal or family history of aneurysms. Inversion does not always mean full inversion – many benefits of inversion therapy, e.g. relieving vertebral disc pressure, can be obtained with partial inversion (Figure 27.4). A commercial inversion table, or an inexpensive slant board may be helpful to a patient willing to innovate at home but not all patients will be inclined to try out something like this on their own and at their own risk.

References

Christensen, K.N., Macfarlane, D.F., Pawlina, W., et al. (2015). A conceptual framework for navigating the superficial territories of the face: Relevant anatomic points for the dermatologic surgeon. Clinical Anatomy 29(2): 237–246.

Davies, C. and Davies, A. (2013). The Trigger Point Therapy Workbook: Your Self-Treatment Guide for Pain Relief. New Harbinger Publications.

Gach, M.R. (2011). Acupressure's Potent Points: A Guide to Self-Care for Common Ailments. Random House Publishing Group.

Shah, J.P., Danoff, J.V., Desai, M.J. et al. (2008 Jan). Biochemicals associated with pain and inflammation are elevated in sites near to and remote from active myofascial trigger points. Archives of Physical Medicine and Rehabilitation 89 (1): 16–23.

Simons, D.G., Travell, J.G., and Simons, L.S. (1999). Travell & Simons' Myofascial Pain and Dysfunction, vol. 2. Lippincott Williams & Wilkins.

Therapies that activate descending pain pathways are essential to patient success in managing chronic pain and include meditation, vocational engagement, empathetic support, distraction, video, music, and sleep optimization. In order to maximize a patient's success against chronic pain, multiple descending modulation therapies should be utilized simultaneously. Sometimes patients "forget" how effective the descending pain pathways can be, but picture an athlete or warrior engaged in goal-directed activity with complete focus – even the pain of a serious injury may not be perceived until hours later when their descending pain suppression abates. While it may not be possible to completely dull all pain, it is possible to benefit from descending modulation and to experience extended periods of substantive relief.

Meditation is perhaps the most extensively studied self-directed descending modulation therapy (Figure 28.1). Developed over millennia, mindfulness mediation demonstrates potent pain-relieving effects and numerous beneficial physiological changes that mitigate chronic pain long-term. Patients may be reluctant to try mindfulness, especially if work and home demands seem overwhelming. If so, it may be helpful to "start small": have the patient agree to spend three minutes a day mindfully breathing. Show them how to install a breathing or meditation app on their phone, note the plan for three minutes daily in their visit instructions and make sure to ask them about progress and barriers at the next visit. Engage in "change talk" around mindfulness – acquiring a mindfulness habit is just that, a new habit. The techniques that work for tobacco cessation are the same methods that can coax patients toward consistent mindfulness. Linked to ACT (Chapter 26), mindfulness not only slows breathing, lowers blood pressure, and reduced stress responses, it will ultimately lead the patient to a state of disentangling their sense of self from the experience of pain – i.e. reaching a state of: "I may not control my pain, but I am not my pain." Mindfulness should be discussed with every patient with chronic pain, even people with life-limiting illness can benefit from mindfulness.

Vocational engagement is a profound form of self-directed pain mitigation that should be discussed with every patient (Figure 28.2) The power of purpose to reduce the impact of uncontrolled chronic pain is almost unparalleled, engagement in finding meaning and purpose can grow naturally from a conversation about what the patient values, as you develop a patient-focused pain self-management plan through motivational interviewing techniques (Frankl 1996; Miller and Rollnick 2013). Vocational engagement does not only mean work-related activity – a meaningful hobby, volunteer work, advocacy, or commitment to family or friends all generate positive focus and the potential for "flow." It must be highly meaningful and not lead the patient to over-extend themselves to the extent that pain flares are frequent and limit progress in therapy.

Empathetic support has been recognized as beneficial in some patients with chronic pain and less useful in others. Women especially may benefit from empathetic engagement, e.g., Doulas in the birthing room. Some clinical studies have not replicated the effects of empathy, but it is a personal choice and for many patients intensely helpful. Make sure to ask your patient about their preferences if painful procedures are anticipated.

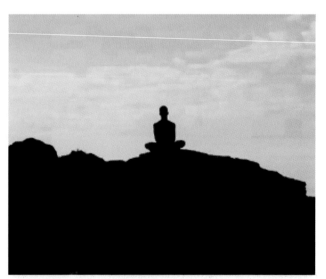

Figure 28.1 Meditation – evidence supports the use of mindfulness-based stress reduction medication techniques. Source: Felipe (Aladim) Hadler/ Free images

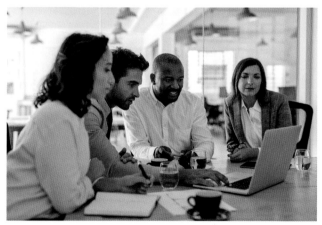

Figure 28.2 Vocational engagement – engaging in meaningful and purposeful activities is associated with less pain. Source: mavoimages/ Adobe Stock Photos

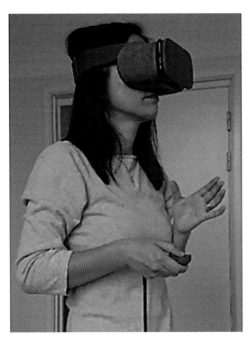

Figure 28.3 Video games and virtual may help reduce stress and pain, however, prolonged sitting and physical activity may be harmful. Source: Garcia-Bonete, M.-J. et al (2019). © John Wiley & Sons.

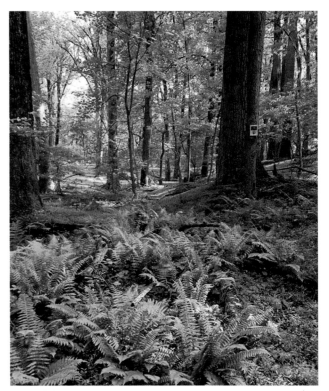

Figure 28.4 Connecting with nature is very therapeutic for some.

Distraction accesses the descending pain modulation system, like empathetic engagement, it is variably effective. Children are often highly responsive to distraction, and it is common for distraction to be used for the management of transient, minor pain, e.g., uncomplicated venipuncture.

Video games can provide pain relief in some settings (Figure 28.3). Not all patients exhibit strong pain modulation in response to video games, e.g., women may be less response to this than men. Video games cannot be played continuously and may interfere with productivity in school or perturb circadian rhythms. Finally, video games are typically played when seated and sedentary, states with long-term negative effects on physiological defenses against pain, and interfering with conditioning and physical activity goals.

Listening to music can engage the descending pain modulation system. Tastes in music are diverse so it is best to avoid specific recommendations, but prescribing scheduled listening, to music that is meaningful or relaxing, can reduce pain. Music listening can be a pleasurable activity that involves minimal cost and is easily integrated into a patient's daily routine. Include music in rescue plans for moderate-to-severe pain flares.

Outdoor exposure "forest bathing" is helpful for some (Figure 28.4).

Sleep is a mandatory every day and yet most of us don't know enough about how to the best night's sleep. For patients with acute or chronic pain, sleep may be especially difficult to obtain in sufficient quantity. Evidence from preclinical studies suggests

that even minor amounts of pain can seriously interfere with good sleep quality in laboratory animals. Good sleep depends on optimizing pain control to the extent safely possible and removing all barriers to sleeping well. Far too many people use computers, cell phones, and televisions until late in the evening – the light emissions of video screens are clearly proven to suppress normal circadian rhythms and this must be discussed with patients during counseling for pain self-management, see Chapter 16 for an overview. Finally, many adults are living with excessive body mass and this is a risk for sleep apnea, a highly prevalent cause of impaired sleep quality, potentially effecting as many as 25% of adult males.

In summary, utilizing treatments that influence descending modulation of pain and engaging patients in as many of these as possible mitigates pain. Most of these therapies have no problematic side effects, other than the cost of time and effort to acquire new and healthier habits.

References

Frankl, V.E. (1959). Man's Search for Meaning: An Introduction to Logotherapy. Boston, MA: Beacon Press.

Miller, W.R. and Rollnick, S. (2013). Motivational Interviewing, Helping People Change, 3e. New York: Guilford Press.

Acute and chronic pain are distinguished primarily by duration (time) but other distinctions include impact, behaviors, and types of pain involved. In defining chronic pain, many favor a fixed-time definition, i.e., pain lasting "more than three months". By contrast, a mechanism-based definition, i.e., pain lasting "longer than the time expected for ordinary healing" holds certain appeal.

Patients typically do not benefit from being labeled with "chronic pain": it is often a pejorative label. Sometimes, patients interpret "chronic" to mean "permanent," increasing pain perpetuation through a cycle of excessive focus on pain. Indeed, excessive pain focusing, to the exclusion of attention to rehabilitative gains is problematic; this does not mean that asking briefly about a pain score is counter-productive. Rather, a pain score reflects the patient's perception, it should be noted but does not need to dominate the entire discussion – ask *how* the patient is doing and *what* they accomplish each day despite living with pain. Chronic pain is useful as a label when recognition transforms care and recruits appropriate resources.

Although each person heals from acute injury at "their own pace," time for healing depends on the tissue and type of injury, Figure 29.1. For example, mild muscle strain heals in days; while a ligamentous tear may never heal completely – causing persistent pain and the inability to accomplish certain movements – unless the tear is surgically repaired. This is not chronic pain as a primary condition of chronic pain but is rather chronic pain secondary to another problem – changes in the pain system, such as sensitization and trigger points may nonetheless follow. Even after a mechanical defect is repaired, some changes can linger or persist – the expectation for most patients is that eventually and with proper therapeutic management, the pain will settle and the function of the pain processing system will normalize. Patients often look to healthcare providers, the "professionals in the room," to establish expected outcomes. Whether psychological or physiological, the effect of establishing generally positive expectations can be life-altering for patients. We don't abandon them on the "pain journey," we remain with them, in spirit and actuality; seeking out effective

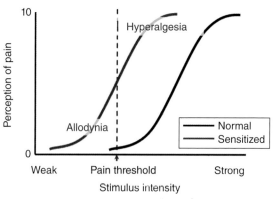

Figure 29.2 In chronic pain, allodynia and hyperalgesia are more prevalent and indicate persistent changes in pain processing. (See also Chapter 3).

therapies, utilizing the knowledge and skill available to us, smoothing the path back to health.

Pain processing in the nervous system is dynamic – extreme (or mild) pain events can be followed by substantive changes in the pain processing system that ultimately result in an increase in the lived pain experience and disablement. Hyperalgesia and allodynia are associated with chronic pain and stand in distinction to "eudynia" or normative pain sensing, Figure 29.2. Allodynia is pain experienced in response to a normally nonpainful stimulus. An example of this is the feeling that warm water provokes when poured over skin that has been recently burned. Whereas cold water relieves the feeling of the burn, warm water, which is normally not painful at all, provokes a highly painful perceived sensation. The feeling of normally comfortable shoes pressing on a newly acquired blister is another example. Hyperalgesia is more intense pain experienced in response to a stimulus that is normally painful. An example of this would be the degree of pain experienced when accidentally falling a second time on a scraped knee – what would normally hurt, hurts way worse if a pre-existing inflamed area is present. In the setting of pain research, we often observe that pain increases as the strength of the noxious stimulus increases – like eating a super-hot chili pepper burns longer and stronger than a mild pepper. This translates into a stimulus-response curve: the stimulus, to some degree, elicits a predictable response. The challenge with pain is individuals vary a lot (interindividual variability). For any particular person however, stimulus-response curves are fairly stable, except when there is an underlying episodic pain condition, like migraine.

Another important difference between acute and chronic pain is "pain behavior." In acute pain, behavior is usually prominent and telegraphs the need for help (see Biopsychosocial model, Chapter 8). This behavior may be suppressible, e.g. in combat. For years, physiologists knew that pain fibers connect directly to motor neurons (in the spinal cord); in the early 1990s, researchers found pain fibers projecting to brain centers usually associated with motor

Pain at three months – is it chronic?

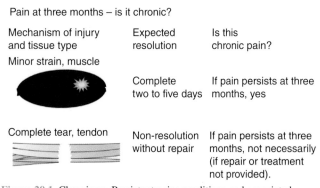

Mechanism of injury and tissue type	Expected resolution	Is this chronic pain?
Minor strain, muscle	Complete two to five days	If pain persists at three months, yes
Complete tear, tendon	Non-resolution without repair	If pain persists at three months, not necessarily (if repair or treatment not provided).

Figure 29.1 Chronic vs. Persistent pain: conditions and associated recovery time frames.

Pain Medicine at a Glance, First Edition. Beth B. Hogans.
© 2022 John Wiley & Sons Ltd. Published 2022 by John Wiley & Sons Ltd.

functions; suggesting that pain behaviors, acutely, are hardwired (Chudler and Dong 1995). People are wired to respond protectively – withdrawing from pain and responding reflexively to maintain balance. In people with chronic pain, these behaviors may not persist. There is evidence that people living with chronic pain have atrophy in brain areas associated with that part of the body where pain manifests. Much remains to be explained but based on multiple lines of research: people living with chronic pain may not demonstrate behaviors that let you know how much pain they are experiencing. For this reason, we need to hear and acknowledge a patient's lived experience of pain.

Finally, it is important to mention that nociceptive pain is less prominent but not nonexistent in patients with chronic pain; inflammatory and neuropathic pain forms are common in patients with persistent pain (Figure 29.3). As noted above, when a mechanical disturbance persists, i.e. unrepaired muscle tear, nociceptive pain may occur with each mechanically disadvantageous movement; there might also be inflammatory and neuropathic pain if the muscle tear lead to structural malpositioning and nerve compression. Genuine curiosity and open inquiry will help healthcare providers recognize that persistent pain is an important clue that perhaps one hasn't yet understood all that is wrong with the patient.

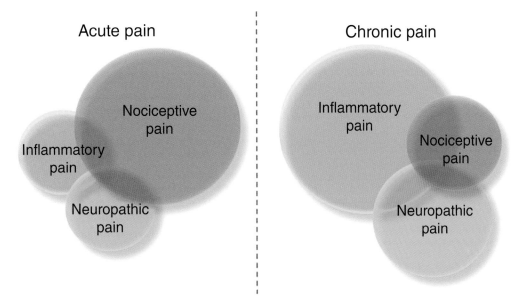

Figure 29.3 Acute vs. Chronic pain: how pain types shift in importance between acute and chronic pain presentations. In acute pain, nociceptive pain is more prevalent, in chronic pain, inflammatory pain predominates.

Reference

Chudler, E.H. and Dong, W.K. (1995). The role of the basal ganglia in nociception and pain. Pain 60 (1): 3–38. https://doi.org/10.1016/0304-3959(94)00172-b.

Surgical and procedural pain (SPP) control is essential for modern surgical and medical care. The control of pain is essential for optimal recovery. Stress responses to surgery are a complicating factor in perioperative pain management, and the relationship with pain is bidirectional: stress makes pain control more challenging, and pain increases physiological and psychological stress, Table 30.1. Controlling pain in the periprocedural and perioperative setting impacts millions of patients annually, but with protocols for multimodal analgesia pre-, intra-, and postoperatively, and evidence-based enhanced recovery programs, outcomes are much improved.

Surgery is very common in the U.S. and around the globe – many surgical procedures are performed in order to reduce pain and improve function. The most common surgical procedures (aside from maternal/neonatal care) are knee and hip surgeries, being the first and second most common, with spine fusion and spinal laminectomy being the fourth and fifth most common, Table 30.2. All of these surgeries will be performed on patients for whom pain is a major symptom. Preoperative pain control is important and has a major impact on outcomes. Because the volume of surgeries performed numbers in the millions, and because pain is a key determinant of outcome, a complex system of quality improvement has evolved to address perioperative care, including pain control; this system is referred to as the Enhance Recovery After Surgery (ERAS) system (AANA 2020). ERAS provides support and organization to advance perioperative procedures and outcomes. Guidance is available through the Veterans Affairs academic detailing service (Himstreet et al. 2017). As Kehlet noted:

> Enhanced recovery protocols are multidisciplinary, perioperative approaches designed to lessen the body's stress response to surgery (ERAS® Society 2020). The protocols and pathways offer us a menu of small changes that, in the aggregate, can lead to large and demonstrable benefits – especially when these small changes are chosen across the preoperative, intraoperative, and postoperative arenas and then standardized in one's practice. Among the major components of ERAS practices and protocols are limiting preoperative fasting, employing multimodal analgesia, encouraging early ambulation and early postsurgical feeding, and creating culture shift to greater emphasis on patient expectations.

To optimize surgical outcomes, it is necessary to gain control over a very complex system – quality improvement approaches address surgical trauma, stress responses, acute and chronic pain, the role of analgesia, cognition, sleep, cardio pulmonary risks function, mobilization, high risk patients – those with low muscle function and mass preoperatively, and to yield the best possible results (Kehlet 2018).

The control of SPP involves multiple factors: temporal, regional vs. systemic pain control, physiological vs. psychological, patient comorbidity, and specific to the surgery or procedure factors.

It is important to plan for pain control from the preprocedural stage: encourage education, moderate physical activity, and provide preanalgesia as needed, Figure 30.1. Periprocedurally, consider regional analgesia, potentially utilizing nerve block as well as systemic analgesia as needed. Early mobilization, multimodal pain control including multiple oral agents, e.g. acetaminophen plus opioid plus NSAID, operative site chilling, compression, elevation, and use of minimally invasive surgery decreases stress stimulus and reduces the likelihood of nerve transection.

Psychological support includes making the patient well informed about the expectations for mobilization, pain control after surgery, and the criteria for discharge.

It is critically important that pain control is responsive to the needs of the patient to engage in rehabilitation-driven movements, i.e., dynamic pain control. Rest pain and dynamic pain vary from procedure to procedure. In addition, patients are highly variable in terms of pain responses, e.g., pain intensity, catastrophizing in response to pain. There is some evidence that opioids may not be as effective for dynamically evoked pain, and better approaches are needed. Multimodal analgesia is associated with reduced length of stay and lower side effects, but there continues to be variability in terms of the elements included in multimodal analgesia. Regional analgesia is a very valuable opioid-sparing approach (Sasaki 2018). Nonpharmacological pain control – chilling (cryotherapy), compression, support, physical activity, distraction,

Table 30.1 Potential harms and side effects of inadequate pain control in the perioperative period.

Consequence of inadequate pain control	Risks and harms associated with functional impairments
Decreased movement	Increased risk of blood clots, muscle atrophy
Decreased deep inspiration	Increased risk of atelectasis, pneumonia
Decreased sleep	Diminished immune function, impaired concentration and cognition, confusion or delirium
Decreased mood	Unwillingness to participate in rehab activities, increased seeking out of passive pain control options
Increased stress	Poor wound healing

Table 30.2 Number of common U.S. surgical procedures, selected procedures as ranked, excluding maternal and neonatal procedures.

Rank	Operating room procedures (all-listed)	Total number of stays
1	Arthroplasty knee	752 921
2	Hip replacement; total and partial	522 820
4	Spinal fusion	463 111
5	Laminectomy; excision intervertebral disc	438 041

Source: HCUP fast stats, 2014 excluding maternal and neonatal.

Pain Medicine at a Glance, First Edition. Beth B. Hogans.
© 2022 John Wiley & Sons Ltd. Published 2022 by John Wiley & Sons Ltd.

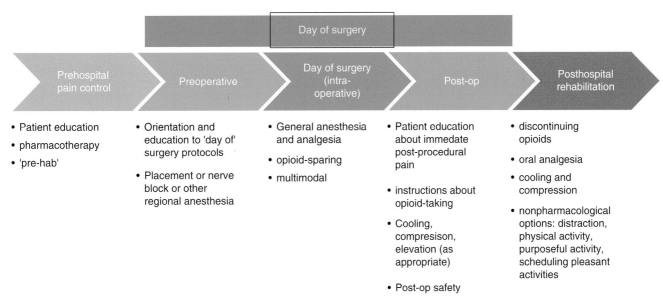

Figure 30.1 Flow diagram for enhanced recovery after surgery protocols. Adapted from AANA (2020).

Is diabetes or obesity present?

Is there preoperative opioid exposure?

What are realistic expectations for physical activity?

What comorbidities impact rehabilitation potential?

Figure 30.2 Prevalent factors that impact outcomes.

and psychological preparation and support can and should be utilized. Control of inflammatory responses is critically important as inflammation increases pain intensity and persistence – nerve block, consistent chilling, elevation, and compression can all contribute to abating inflammation and further improve pain control. Finally, sleep disturbances must be avoided, for example, there is a loss of REM sleep when patients are hospitalized; with ERAS protocols, emphasis on returning patients to home rapidly can contribute to avoiding sleep deprivation which would ultimately increase pain perception.

The use of oral opioids for SPP has undergone dramatic reappraisal recently and the number of opioids prescribed after surgery has declined dramatically. For many surgeries, a much smaller number of tablets, at lower strength, is now prescribed, and patients mostly tolerate this very well. Most patients have a rapid decline in pain following limb surgery so that opioids are most helpful for the first two to five days. Occasionally a patient will have more intense or persistent pain, in which event, the surgical team will need to be aware of this, consider in person vs. remote assessment, and make an informed decision about next steps, Figure 30.2. Some surgeries, such as extensive spinal surgery, may have a more protracted course of pain recovery. The purpose of pain medication is not to eliminate all pain, but rather reduce pain to tolerable levels and to compliment the other therapies that mitigate pain, including intermittent activity and rest, cryotherapy, compression, and elevation as well as others noted above.

References

AANA (American Association of Nurse Anesthetists) (2020). Enhanced recovery after surgery. https://www.aana.com/practice/clinical-practice-resources/enhanced-recovery-after-surgery (accessed 5 July 2020).

ERAS® Society (2020). The mission of the ERAS Society is to develop perioperative care and to improve recovery through research, education, audit and implementation of evidence-based practice. https://erassociety.org/about/history/ (accessed 2 July 2020).

HCUP (2014). HCUP fast stats, 2014 excluding maternal and neonatal. https://hcup-us.ahrq.gov/faststats/NationalProceduresServlet?year1=2014&characteristic1=0&included1=0&year2=2008&characteristic2=54&included2=1&expansionInfoState=hide&dataTablesState=hide&definitionsState=hide&exportState=hide.

Kehlet, H. (2018). Post-operative pain and rehabilitation. Plenary presentation. Learning Objectives: Provide an updated review on postoperative pain guidelines, Understand the requirement for a procedure-specific approach, Understand the importance of integrating postoperative pain management into an enhanced recovery program. IASP Pain World Congress, Boston, MA.

Himstreet, J., Popish, S.J., Wells, D.L. et al. (2017). Acute Pain Management. Meeting the Challenges. (Provider Education Guide) IB&P Number: IB 10-998; P96864 VA Academic Detailing Service. Washington DC. https://www.pbm.va.gov/PBM/AcademicDetailingService/Documents/Academic_Detailing_Educational_Material_Catalog/Pain_Provider_AcutePainProviderEducationalGuide_IB10998.pdf (accessed 30 December 2020).

Sasaki, K. (2018). Master class: implementing enhanced recovery protocols for gynecologic surgery. https://www.mdedge.com/obgyn/article/156945/pain/implementing-enhanced-recovery-protocols-gynecologic-surgery (accessed 5 July 2020).

Musculoskeletal pain is the most common and disabling form of pain globally. Musculoskeletal pain increases substantively with age but is less diagnosed late in life. Women experience musculoskeletal pain more often than men. Major principles can guide diagnosis and therapy of musculoskeletal pain.

Musculoskeletal structures are variably innervated; under conditions of chronic stress and recurrent injury, the innervating nerves can shift to a pain-sensing phenotype. Even 15 years ago, it was not known that recurrently strained and damaged intervertebral discs are gradually penetrated with pain-sensing nerve fibers. Notably, few football players can continue their professional sports careers indefinitely, typically due to severe low back and joint pain. The musculoskeletal system responds dynamically to strain; therefore, it is critical for people to prepare correctly when physical demands are anticipated. Essentially the entire range of pain-associated musculoskeletal conditions responds to "comprehensive" pain management approaches that proactively incorporate nonpharmacological approaches balanced with pharmacological therapies, note that recover times vary by structure, Figure 31.1.

Medications used for musculoskeletal conditions have risks. All widely available treatments have lethal potential. Acetaminophen, despite generally excellent safety, can cause lethal liver damage in persons with hepatic impairment, alcoholism, or through overdose. NSAIDs result in many gastrointestinal bleeding events, including fatal events, more commonly in older adults. Opioids can be lethal and should not be combined with benzodiazepines, muscle relaxants, or respiratory suppressants such as alcohol, drugs of abuse; careful monitoring in those with respiratory compromise is mandatory. All persons receiving opioids require screening and monitoring (Himstreet et al. 2017).

Interventional techniques are widely used for painful musculoskeletal conditions. Although it is always hoped that an intervention will be curative, not atypically, a series of injections would be necessary to maintain symptomatic control. It is absolutely crucial to recognize that each injection or procedure creates a window of opportunity for the patient to engage in physical activity and physical therapy – potentially correcting maladaptive movement patterns. Prepare patients for the reality that the opportunity must not be wasted – once pain returns, they will be waiting dolefully for the next injection and unable to fully engage in the exercises and activities essential for long-term functional restoration.

Physical therapy should be part of almost every treatment plan for pain of musculoskeletal origin. This may be a basic as offering simple guidance on general activity or selected stretching exercises well-known to the provider, or may extend to a course of therapy visits. Physical therapists (PTs) are typically well-informed about musculoskeletal conditions. Primary care practitioners can benefit from close collaboration with a knowledgeable physical therapist who may enhance diagnosis and advance treatment. Patients rely on their trusted primary care provider but a great physical therapist can create a whole new outlook for a patient. PTs play a vital role at a critical juncture – encouraging activity and recalibrating expectations for healthy activity. For older adults, physical therapy becomes even more important, preventing muscle loss and falls.

Pain self-management is critically important for patients with musculoskeletal conditions. Musculoskeletal pain typically involves both inflammatory and nociceptive mechanisms. Nociceptive pain can arise from barely perceptible microtraumas or minor events that the patient has trouble recalling, but which the

Condition	Recovery time frame
Muscle strain: pulled muscle	Two to four days
Muscle tear	One to three weeks, may require surgery
Muscle cramps	Minutes, may require workup
Trigger points/muscle spasms	Resolve slowly w/o treatment
Tendonitis	Months
Ligamentous strain	May require ergonomic adjust.
Ligamentous tear	May heal very slowly
Soft tissue contusion	Days if not serious
Spondylolisthesis (incl. S-I joint)	Intermittent severe pain
Joint arthritis	Permanent with flairs
Fracture	Severe three to seven days, then six wks
Bone contusion	Days-weeks, varies with severity
Disc herniation	Six to eight weeks, may need surgery
Disc tear	One to three months`
Disc-vertebral dysfunction	Months with flairs
Nerve compression	Chronic unless relieved

Figure 31.1 Chronic vs. Persistent pain: conditions and associated recovery time frames.

Pain Medicine at a Glance, First Edition. Beth B. Hogans.
© 2022 John Wiley & Sons Ltd. Published 2022 by John Wiley & Sons Ltd.

Nonpharmacological management of pain:
useful for musculoskeletal pain

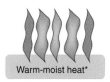

Warm-moist heat*

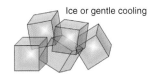

Ice or gentle cooling

Acupressure or trigger point massage

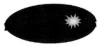

Patient and environmental factors

Dr. Ann algesia
Rx:
Ergonomic evaluation
Physical therapy
Limit lifting: <10 lbs, two weeks

*Heat is not effective for neuropathy

Figure 31.2 Selected nonpharmacological therapies for musculoskeletal pain conditions.

body responds to with pain. This nature of pain should be drawn out in discussion with the patient, the provider can suggest a trial of 20-minute ice-pack applications, perhaps alternating with a heating pad, Figure 31.2. Highlight for the patient that when they find that ice is helpful, it is essential, as not moving is not an option. Physical therapists almost always apply ice for 10 minutes after PT – ice blocks pain and prevents repeated microtrauma and inflammation. The value of moderate daily activity cannot be over-stressed – it is possible to expand activity gradually, for patients with chronic pain, this may involve small incremental increases (10%) in activity each week.

Diagnostically, it is essential to recognize **musculoskeletal pain patterns** i.e. monoarticular, polyarticular, muscle-related, enthesiopathy-like. A patient's symptoms should prompt evaluation of specific body parts to identify key features: tenderness to palpation, edema, discoloration, thermal change, or pain with movement (dolor, tumor, rubor, calor). Generally, monoarticular conditions may require evaluation by orthopedists; polyarticular, or enthesiopathy-related conditions evaluation by rheumatology; and muscle-related conditions by neuromuscular-neurologists.

Consequences of musculoskeletal pain include sleep disturbance, mood interference, cognitive impairment, brain atrophy, focal muscle loss, and increased falls. Even a minor amount of pain-related nerve signals can prevent deep-phase restorative sleep. Address this by offering multiple strategies to optimize night-time pain control (when day-time strategies of distraction, vocational engagement, moderate physical activities, etc. are not possible). How often have you noticed someone express anger, anguish, or frustration in response to articular pain – pain is intimately related to mood but the impacts of pain on mood are universally negative. Cognitively, musculoskeletal pain limits sustained concentration – it is essentially an interrupt signal in the "train of thought." Related to this, there is terrifying evidence that brain atrophy results from chronic pain, what is not known yet is whether alleviating this pain ultimately leads to a restoration of brain structures or whether this does not ever happen. What is often overlooked however is the profound loss of muscle mass that occurs in certain muscles following articular injury: knee injury for example can produce marked atrophy of the quadriceps in the anterior thigh – partially due to involuntary reflex-driven suppression of muscle activity. Finally, for older adults, musculoskeletal pain increases falls. Whether from avoidant movement or weakness, the risks are severe as an ill-timed fall can lead to death or permanent loss of independence.

Reference

Himstreet, J., Popish, S.J., Wells, D.L. et al. (2017). Acute Pain Management. Meeting the Challenges. (Provider Education Guide) IB&P Number: IB 10-998; P96864 VA Academic Detailing Service. Washington DC. https://www.pbm.va.gov/PBM/AcademicDetailingService/Documents/Academic_Detailing_Educational_Material_Catalog/Pain_Provider_AcutePainProviderEducationalGuide_IB10998.pdf (accessed 30 December 2020).

Orofacial syndromes involve face and oral structures, distinct from headache. Orofacial pain can arise from nociceptive, inflammatory, and neuropathic pain mechanisms. Anatomical factors and patterns are essential to understanding these syndromes. Although neuropathic conditions are not the most prevalent, they are highly distressing and challenging to treat, comprising a substantive part of clinical effort. Different forms of orofacial pain require various treatments, but comprehensive treatment is essential (Chapter 16) (Stuhr et al. 2014).

Anatomy and innervation

The face and anterior head are innervated largely by the trigeminal nerve; three divisions: ophthalmic, maxillary, and mandibular supply sensation to the upper, middle, and lower face (Figure 32.1). Tongue and oropharynx sensation are supplied by cranial nerves V, VII, IX, and X with the third division of V supplying general sensation of the anterior tongue while VII supplies taste (special sensory), IX supplies both taste and general sensation to the posterior tongue (Figure 32.2). All oral and pharyngeal structures have complex nerve supplies that include somatic sensation, special sense of taste, and autonomic sensory fibers as well. These structures are closely arranged together with other critical structures including eyes and optic nerves, ears and associated structures, and the base of the brain (Sola et al. 2020). In the

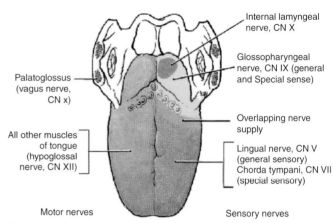

Figure 32.2 Innervation of the tongue.

presence of general symptoms or focal neurological deficits, it may be necessary to consider post-traumatic, infectious, and neoplastic space-occupying lesions, in clinical context.

Common and relevant conditions

Pulpitis, inflammation of the dental pulp, rapidly produces severe nociceptive oral pain. Modern dentistry, through remarkable advances in pain control, means that most general dentists can resolve this pain immediately. Dental sensitivity to heat and cold should prompt one to seek routine dental care, as by the stage of an acute severe pulpitis, it may be too late to forestall the loss of the tooth and the accompanying cost of a crown or implant. Avoidance of sugary beverages and sweets combined with fluoride, maintenance dental treatments, and conscientious routine brushing and flossing are the best preventatives. It is remarkable that chemical nerve destruction, typically performed to alleviate the pain of pulpitis, is completely and immediately effective in relieving what is otherwise a shatteringly severe pain, and only very rarely results in any development of a chronic pain syndrome, many dentists may never see a single patient with neuropathic pain arising from uncomplicated dental caries (Figure 32.3). Complex dental problems can be a cause of chronic orofacial pain, this should be considered in the differential diagnosis when appropriate.

Temporomandibular joint disorder (TMD) is a chronic painful syndrome associated with pain that is worse on movement of the temporomandibular joint. When more than mild, this syndrome can greatly impair normal function as the person with TMD may have difficulty with normal speaking and eating activities. Dental evaluation and symptomatic treatment with NSAIDs, oral rest and thermal therapies may be helpful for milder forms, early dental involvement is also important. More severe forms may require recruitment of additional therapeutic modalities such as cognitive-behavioral therapy (CBT) and biofeedback. Patients with chronic TMD may be at risk for

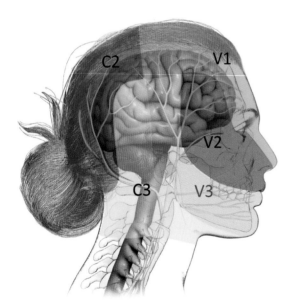

Figure 32.1 Segmental (dermatomal) innervation of face and head, lateral view. 'V' is the 5th cranial nerve with three branches. 'C' is the cervical spinal level as indicated. Nerves in figure are motor nerves; sensation is mediated by sensory components of the trigeminal nerve (V) and the 2nd and 3rd dorsal cervical rami. The first cervical level does not have a sensory dermatome. Source: Pixdesign123/Adobe Stock.

Pain Medicine at a Glance, First Edition. Beth B. Hogans.
© 2022 John Wiley & Sons Ltd. Published 2022 by John Wiley & Sons Ltd.

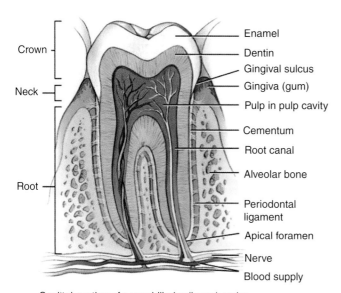

Sagittal section of a manidibular (lower) molar

Figure 32.3 Pulpitis typically resolves rapidly and completely with denervation of the tooth. Source: © 2009, John Wiley & Sons.

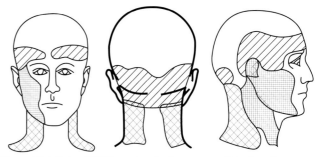

Figure 32.4 Pain of TMD can involve large areas of the face. Source: Stuhr et al. (2014). Reproduced with permission of Taylor & Francis Ltd.

other chronic inflammatory conditions, including inflammatory bowel syndrome, through mechanisms that are as yet poorly understood.

Trigeminal Neuralgia (TGN) involves deeply distressing neuropathic pain of the trigeminal nerve (Figure 32.4). Lancinating (sword-like) or electrical (shocking jolt-like) pain develops insidiously, sometimes without clear precipitant. Some TGN arises from nerve compression from nearby skull-base blood vessels, others have observed very high rates of herpes virus in perineural fluid. Typically, carbamazepine controls symptoms, oxcarbazepine may be an alternative. Sometimes interventional or surgical therapies work, but not as first-line therapy (Dimitroulis 2018). Comprehensive management of TGN includes nonpharmacological therapies (Gauer and Semidey 2015). Many patients with neuropathic pain syndromes, including TGN, find that pain levels increase when stress flares and remit when self-management strategies are fully engaged and general stress is mitigated.

Ocular Postherpetic neuralgia can affect the cornea – the result is unreal amounts of pain as the cornea is very densely innervated with pain-sensing nerve fibers. Ocular PHN can primarily involve neuropathic pain compounded by dry eye and other autonomic changes leading to chronic corneal damage creating a wretched combination of neuropathic, inflammatory, and nociceptive pain. These patients may require detailed and interlocking pharmacological and nonpharmacological therapies. For these patients, it may be especially beneficial to refer them to a sleep-specializing clinical psychologist, ideally someone who is empathetic to and knowledgeable about patients with chronic pain. Close communication with the patient, pharmacist, clinical psychologist, neurologist, and ophthalmologist will be helpful. Standard procedures such as having the patient keep a pain calendar will be very helpful as treatment optimization will likely require a series of iterative adjustments to treatment and the pain intensity and quality information in the calendar will be valuable in making informed decisions. Compassion is essential, it must be woven together with careful attention to making good therapeutic choices. As this is absolutely a chronic condition with a long recovery cycle, opioids may not be an especially ideal choice given that the efficacy of opioids against pain declines with time – other medications that do not manifest effect tolerance may be a better choice.

Burning mouth syndrome is a relatively rare syndrome that affects more women than men, developing often in late middle age (National Institute of Dental and Craniofacial Research 2020). Characterized by burning pain, tingling, or distressing numbness in the tongue, soft palate, or other mouth structures, this pain may be unremitting for weeks on end. Therapies include medications, avoidance of irritating substances (tobacco, alcohol, and spicy foods), and comprehensive pain management (Imamura et al. 2019). An appropriate evaluation is needed to ensure that no underlying or complicating conditions exist.

For references, please turn to page 108.

Neck pain is prevalent and often challenging to treat – but when patients and providers collaborate to avoid passive strategies, ('PT over pills'), positive results ensue. Occuring at about 1/5th the rate of low back pain; cervicalgia is often chronic.

Anatomy and innervation

Neck structures include densely packed critical conduits for circulation, respiration, nutrition, and nervous system function, as well as supporting the head. The anterior neck contains major arteries, veins, lymphatics, oropharynx, trachea, thyroid, esophagus, and tongue-base structures (Figure 33.1). Anterior neck pain should prompt screening for space-occupying or infectious processes – with diagnostic testing if necessary. The cervical spinal column (posterior neck) supports and protects the cervical spinal cord through which all nerves pass between brain and body. Spinal muscles, bone, and ligaments subserve movement in multiple directions. Vertebral bodies are near the neck cross-sectional center; the spinal cord is immediately posterior. The spinal cord enlarges cross-sectionally in the areas supplying limb innervation, with corresponding enlargement of the spinal canal. The spinal canal is bounded by vertebral bodies anteriorly, and vertebral pedicles and laminae with numerous ligaments and soft tissues laterally and posteriorly (Figure 33.2). Cervical nerve roots are shorter than lumbosacral roots, horizontally traversing the spinal canal before exiting at neural foramina. Sensory nerve cell bodies reside in dorsal root ganglia that sit in small recesses (neural foraminae) between adjacent vertebral pedicles. Early in

life, these recesses are well-protected and spacious for the ganglia; however, in later life, arthritic enlargement of nearby vertebral and facet joints, leads to compression of ganglia and nerves.

Common and relevant conditions

Although the brain famously "does not feel pain when injured," injury to the posterior (dorsal) and central components of the spinal cord can produce profound diffuse myelopathic pain that resists ordinary pharmacological therapies. In addition, the cervical spine is quite prone to degenerative syndromes of disc herniation, nerve compression, arthritic degeneration, and disc strain or tears. These syndromes are also intensely painful, typically more localizable, but are also resistant to basic remedies. Although less common, thoracic disc injury and thoracic nerve compression, e.g vertebral collapse from osteoporosis or trauma, can have substantial negative impacts on breathing, decreasing minute volumes and oxygenation through reflex respiratory splinting. Major causes of neck, cervical, and thoracic pain include nociceptive, inflammatory, and neuropathic conditions, especially cervical whiplash, facet joint osteoarthritis, cervical radiculopathy, and diabetic mononeuropathy. There are many causes of neck, cervical, and thoracic pain that require investigation; diagnostic tests, including imaging, should be pursued when history and exam findings suggest relevant processes. It is not uncommon for infectious diseases such as

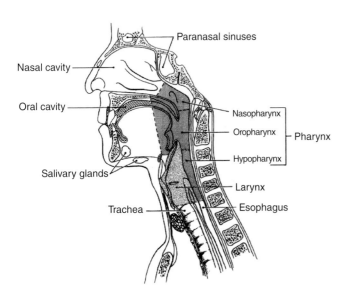

Figure 33.1 Sagittal view of the neck, illustrating structures of anterior neck.

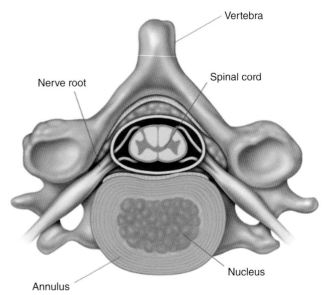

Figure 33.2 Cross-sectional view of cervical spinal column, muscles removed. Note the relative short length of the cervical roots and the location of the cervical dorsal root ganglia, between the vertebral disc and the fact joints.

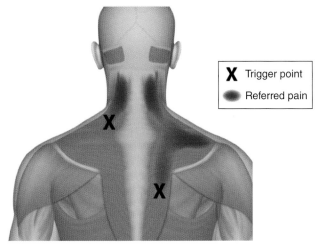

Figure 33.3 Trigger points in the shoulder girdle contribute to neck pain, palpation for trigger points is an important part of examining patients with neck pain.

| X | Trigger point |
| • | Referred pain |

epidural abscesses, Lyme disease, and tuberculosis, or for inflammatory conditions such as multiple sclerosis to present with cervical or thoracic symptoms.

Cervical whiplash is a common sequela of accelerative injuries (rear-end motor vehicle accidents). For decades, cervical whiplash was dismissed as "soft tissue" injury ascribed to litigants pursuing insurance company payouts. Soft tissue injury is visualizable on MRI: healing times vary with the soft tissue involved and injury severity. Muscles, even minimally injured, can produce intense focal pain, typically resolving by five days if the provoking activity is avoided. Muscle tears take significantly longer to heal, tendon strains, sprains, and tears take longer with successively severe injury. Ligamentous injuries may never fully heal and can result in pain either through reflex muscle spasms producing profound and persistent pain, or aberrant patterns of motion leading to accelerated wear and chronic pain. In addition, in the cervical spine, nerve roots are vulnerable to compression, further perpetuating pain. Research previously focused on nonmodifiable factors such as age, gender, and socioeconomic status as predicting chronic pain, but recent studies show that intense pain, early after injury, predicts whiplash persistence (Sarrami et al. 2017). Finally, there is potential for central pain upregulation (sensitization). Comprehensive management with (Chapter 16) care coordination should be fairly aggressive seeking rapid resolution (Tobbackx et al. 2013). Pharmacological strategies often employ skeletal muscle relaxants; however, these must not be combined with CNS depressants, e.g. opioids, alcohol.

Facet joint osteoarthritis common affects older adults. Facet joints are true synovial joints and other treatments used for osteoarthritis may be effective. Located lateral to the midline, posteriorly; chronic strain enlarges facet joints potentially compressing the adjacent nerve root(s) and contributing to central canal stenosis. The cervical facet joints are more horizontally oriented (permitting rotational movement) than are thoracic or lumbar facet joints. Potentially injured by accidents or maladaptive movements; facet joint pain is aching to sharp, and often chronic or episodic in nature. Management strategies include: PT – strengthening and range of motion, thermal therapies, treatment of relevant trigger points – and coordinated pharmacotherapy (Figure 33.3).

Cervical radiculopathy often severely painful and debilitating, potentially includes nociceptive, inflammatory, and neuropathic components, with pain that radiates from neck into arm. Disc protrusions, tears, and herniations, and facet joint hypertrophy contribute to nerve compression. Radiculopathy may be resistant to simple treatments – coordinated comprehensive management including multiple pharmacological agents and interventional approaches. Cervical epidural steroid injections are riskier than lumbar epidural steroid injections. Other therapeutic approaches including physical therapy, traction, focal muscle relaxation, trigger point approaches, or iontophoresis may be worth pursuing first. Communicate with local physical therapists to ensure they are knowledgeable and engaged as they treat patients with cervical pain.

Diabetic mononeuropathy is a cause of focal neuropathic pain potentially arising in any peripheral nerve but occurrence in thoracic vertebral nerves is not uncommon. Essentially a nerve microinfarct, prevention through scrupulous diabetic control is preferred as once neuropathic pain is established, complex comprehensive management is needed.

References

Sarrami, P et al. (2017). Factors predicting outcome in whiplash injury: a systematic meta-review of prognostic factors. J Ortho Traum 18: 9–16.

Tobbackx, Y et al. (2013). Does acupuncture activate endogenous analgesia in chronic whiplash-associated disorders? EJP 17:279–89.

Although not as common as back and leg pain, arm pain is highly prevalent and disabling. In older adults, shoulder pain is the fifth most common cause of pain, persisting unless actively treated. Rotator cuff injuries, hand OA, and nerve compression (CTS and ulnar nerve) are common.

Arm pain is surprisingly disabling; vocational activity places many demands on the arms. Some basic general principles are useful: (i) proximal arm pain, e.g. shoulder pain, is often unilateral whereas distal pain is very often bilateral, (ii) proximal arm pain is most often musculoskeletal, e.g. rotator cuff, while distal pain has a broad differential diagnosis including focal processes and systemic illnesses, e.g., carpal tunnel syndrome and rheumatoid arthritis, and (iii) arm pain diagnosis often relies on "expert pattern recognition" in part because are innervation and pain processing are complex. To preserve essential function, referral for expert care is often indicated for acute hand and arm pain (Brushart 2011).

Anatomy and innervation

The arm consists of the shoulder girdle, the arm proper (shoulder to elbow); the forearm (elbow to wrist); the wrist, and the hand (Figure 34.1). Three large nerves, the median, the ulnar, and the radial, enter the arm by way of the brachial plexus which arises from spinal root levels C5 to T1. The median nerve has a protected course

in the (upper) arm then passes through forearm anteriorly to enter the palm through the carpal tunnel in the mid-anterior wrist (Figure 34.2). Providing sensation and motor function to the thumb, it is essential for normal hand function (LeBlond and Donald 2014). The ulnar nerve is also fairly protected in the arm, but is vulnerable to stretch and compression injury as it rounds the corner on the lower (medial) elbow, it then passes through the forearm to enter the hand on the side of the "little" finger (Figure 34.3). The radial nerve is vulnerable to compression against posterior humerus in the arm, the syndromes of "Saturday night palsy" and "Bridegroom's palsy" reflect the

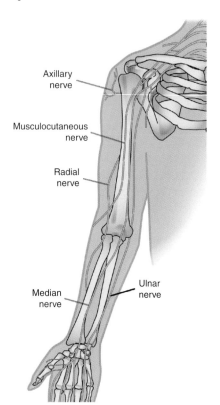

Figure 34.1 Diagram of arm with major nerves: median, ulnar, and radial; illustrating location of brachial plexus.

Axillary nerve

Musculocutaneous nerve

Radial nerve

Median nerve

Ulnar nerve

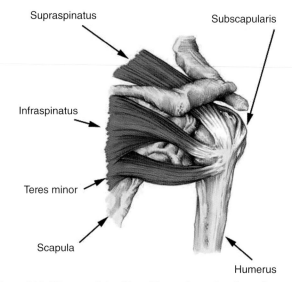

Supraspinatus

Subscapularis

Infraspinatus

Teres minor

Scapula

Humerus

Figure 34.2 Diagram of shoulder with muscles and tendons of rotator cuff.

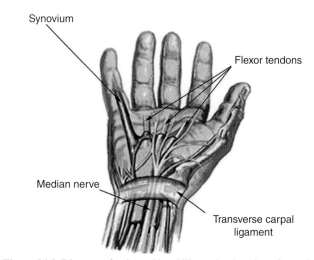

Synovium

Flexor tendons

Median nerve

Transverse carpal ligament

Figure 34.3 Diagram of wrist and hand illustrating location of carpal tunnel compression.

Pain Medicine at a Glance, First Edition. Beth B. Hogans.
© 2022 John Wiley & Sons Ltd. Published 2022 by John Wiley & Sons Ltd.

colorful events provoking damage to this nerve (O'Brien 2010). Otherwise, the radial nerve has a protected course and is often used in nerve conduction studies as a "normal comparison nerve," less often damaged than the median or ulnar nerves.

Common and relevant conditions

Differential diagnosis of arm, shoulder, and hand pain relies heavily on expert pattern recognition, due to the complex innervation and movement patterns (Figure 34.4). Referral for expert evaluation is often warranted due to the implications of loss-of-function for productivity and daily activities. The mechanism-based classification of pain-associated conditions is important for understanding pain in the arm.

Sprain, strain, and fractures are common in the arm, hand, and shoulder girdle. Pain related to acute injury is nociceptive. Prompt first-aid pain control follows the RICE-M model: rest the part, ice the area, compress by placing a splint or compression wrap (ensuring good circulation is preserved), elevate the limb to prevent undue swelling, and medicate for pain control. Opioids should be reserved for major fracture or trauma. Acute injuries vary by age group, with rotator cuff tears and strains being more common in older adults; fractures and sprains occur at any age but are very common in children (Figure 34.5). Prompt expert evaluation and diagnostic testing is often appropriate.

Tendinitis is highly painful inflammatory-related pain. Locations of tendinitis vary but "tennis-elbow" at the lateral epicondyle is classic. Tendinitis can be very painful, treatment refractory, and recurrent. Prevention or very early "aggressive" management are critical. Rest, alone, is often not sufficient – expert management is key. **Hand osteoarthritis** is a chronic inflammatory-type pain-associated hand condition. OA of the thumb base is very common, management often includes referral to occupational therapy for bracing, immobilization, and exercises, e.g. putty. Bouts may recur and once expert evaluation has determined the correct course of action, patient engagement should be encouraged.

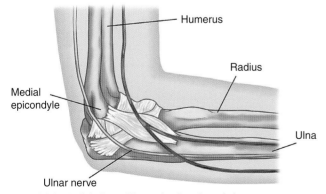

Figure 34.4 Medial elbow, illustrating location of ulnar nerve compressive neuropathy.

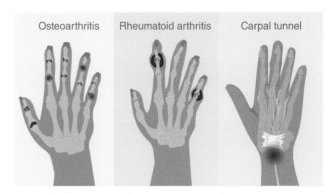

Figure 34.5 Comparison of pain patterns in hand.

Carpal tunnel syndrome is a well-known syndrome of neuropathic pain and weakness that impacts the hand. The pain of carpal tunnel can be a pins-and-needles irritation or a deep aching pain, it can present in the hand or in some patients, radiate up into the forearm. Sometimes pain is not prominent, but despite this nerve damage can lead to weakness. If weakness or muscle atrophy is present, prompt evaluation by an expert is necessary to preserve future function. Atrophy is detected by careful inspection of the thenar eminence of the hand – flattening of the normally plump muscle body, the presence of skin wrinkling, or focal muscle loss all suggest that speedy assessment and resolution are needed. If bothersome pain is present without muscle atrophy, it may be reasonable to provide immobilization, e.g. carpal tunnel splints, while awaiting expert input; care must be taken to ensure that the splint does not impede circulation or add additional compression to the wrist.

Ulnar nerve compression at the elbow is very common (perhaps 50% of adults). Worsened by elbow bending, such as holding a phone or sleeping with arms curled up, ulnar nerve damage can lead to permanent and disabling hand weakness as well as chronic pain in the form of neuropathic hyperalgesia. A quick screen for this involves inspecting the hands visually: if the little finger 'sticks out' from the other fingers rather than 'pointing forwards with the rest of the fingers', this is evidence to suggest that ulnar nerve damage is weakening the muscles that would normally align the little finger with the other digits. **Radiculopathy** (neuropathic pain) discussed in detail in Chapter 32. Thoracic outlet syndrome is another nerve compression syndrome producing arm pain and weakness.

Prompt diagnosis and treatment of arm and hand pain is complex but essential for the preservation of function, referral for expert management is often necessary.

References

Brushart, T.M. (ed.) (2011). Clinical nerve repair and grafting. In: Nerve Repair. Oxford, UK: Oxford University Press.

LeBlond, R. and Brown, D. (2014). DeGowin's Diagnostic Examination, 10 (Lange). McGraw-Hill.

O'Brien, M. (2010). Aids to the Examination of the Peripheral Nervous System 5. Saunders.

Back pain, the most common form of pain, causes years lost to disability globally (Wu et al. 2020). Despite extraordinary prevalence and impact, education and research are limited; clinical myths persist (Mezei et al. 2011). Once "red flags" are excluded (Chapter 36), patients are eager for relief. Recognizing and treating the common forms are addressed here.

For low back pain, the most efficient entry point into diagnosis depends on the key pain features – **location** is the most important diagnostic clue (Murinson 2011). The common low back conditions: muscle strain, ligamentous strain, disc injury, nerve compression (radiculopathy/sciatica), facet joint arthritis, and sacroiliac joint dysfunction typically have characteristic pain patterns (Figure 35.1).

Muscle strain may be the most common cause of low back pain. Sometimes acutely painful, it can resolve quickly, but when the provoking activity persists, e.g. truck driving, housecleaning, pain will continue. Typically off of the midline and aching, burning, or sharp in quality, this pain should respond to cessation of the provoking activity (with maintenance of general activity), and conservative therapies including cold-packs, heating pads, epsom salt baths or compresses, massage, trigger-point therapy, acupuncture, chiropractic, or oral over-the-counter medications. Pain of suspected muscle strain lasting longer than two weeks should prompt further assessment or ergonomic evaluation.

Ligamentous strain is a widespread and generally benign although bothersome cause of low- and mid-back pain. Although ligaments themselves may not be painful, the strain of ligaments from malpositioning and incorrect postures can cause muscle spasms persisting for days afterward. Pain is diffuse, near midline (one or both sides), aching, burning, or sharp in quality, and persistent. Standard therapies provide only transient relief. These patients must have physical therapy to improve posture, and a workplace ergonomic assessment, where available. If occupational support is not available, have someone video or photo the patient at their work-station – then discuss potential problems and engage cooperation with addressing chronic precipitants. Patients with underlying scoliosis may present asymmetrically.

Disc injury varies with age – frank disc herniation occurs more in early midlife when disc are still elastic, where as disc degeneration can be quite painful in later midlife when discs have become sensitized due to ingrowth of pain-sensing nerve fibers following repeated cycles of trauma and healing. Disc injuries may have provoking precipitants but many patients don't identify any, Figure 35.2. The pain is often sharp, in the midline with minor radiation, and can be so much worse with movement that standing and sitting are effectively impossible. The disc takes much longer than muscle to heal, there is limited blood supply. Smoking makes this worse. Because changes in

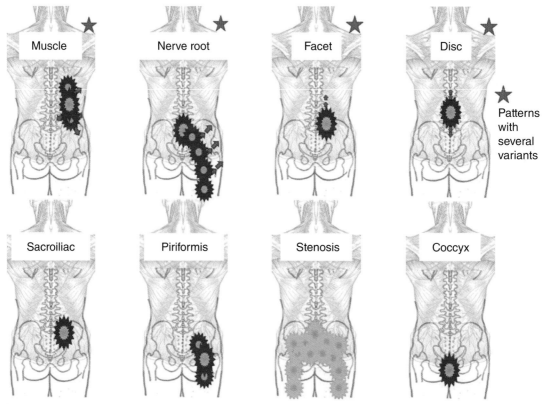

Figure 35.1 Pain patterns often associated with common causes of low back pain – pattern recognition aid.

Pain Medicine at a Glance, First Edition. Beth B. Hogans.

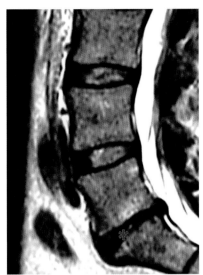

Figure 35.2 Lumbosacral spine sagittal MRI. Degenerated, desiccated disc is marked with an asterisk

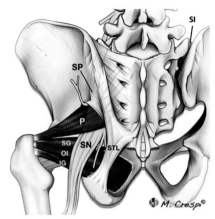

Figure 35.4 Diagram illustrating SI joint in posterior pelvis/lateral low back, note also sciatic nerve and piriformis muscle

position provoke wide swings in disc pressure, normal movement can provoke pain flares. Although one major study reported bedrest was of no help, the detailed data showed pronounced relief of pain during bedrest, that rapidly reversed with the resumption of activity (Vroomen et al. 1999). Because continuous bedrest results in dangerous muscle atrophy, activity is encouraged, to the extent tolerated. Patients *must* attend physical therapy for muscle strengthening complimenting intermittent recumbency as a pain-relieving strategy. Some patients find relief in traction, partial inversion, chiropractic, or back belts – treatments must be individualized to feasibility, fitness, and available therapies. Long-term, physical conditioning prevents reinjury.

Facet joint arthritis is a degenerative joint condition that increases with age, Figure 35.3. Typically associated with para-axial (lateral pain near the spine) pain that is exacerbated with spine extension or backward bending, facet joint arthritis pain is dull, aching, burning, or sharp. It occurs in bouts or chronically. It requires comprehensive

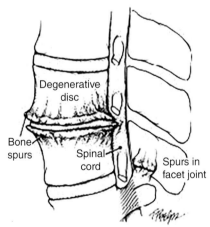

Figure 35.3 Schematic diagram illustrating changes associated with disc degeneration, note also facet OA

For references, see page 108.

pain management with optimization of muscle condition (physical therapy), posture, and integration of moderate daily exercise, sleep hygiene, thermal therapies, and trigger point therapy. Focal topical agents may help, as can chiropractic or traction. Rescue therapy with oral over-the-counter analgesia may be helpful but over reliance pill-taking strategies should be discouraged.

Sacroiliac joint dysfunction is highly prevalent, presenting with disablingly severe lateral "low back" pain, Figure 35.4. Typically at the level of the posterior superior iliac "spine," the pain is so characteristic, it is "localizable by a finger." Ask the patient to point to the most severe pain spot with a single finger; if this is the lateral low back, at the level of the lumbosacral junction, about 3 inches lateral of the midline, then SI joint dysfunction should be suspected. This pain is dull, aching, or burning at rest, but intensely sharp with movements – walking on stairs, stepping off a curb, or arising from a chair. The joint can be repositioned by those qualified in manual therapy (physical therapists, osteopathic physicians, or chiropractors). Repeated cycles of dislocation should be avoided as chronic joint dysfunction resists treatment. Pelvic girdle belts, analgesia, and comprehensive management are useful.

Spondylolisthesis, an overlooked but not uncommon condition, prevalent in older adults, is characterized by generally benign but intensely painful spinal instability. Pain typically occurs in time-limited bouts of disabling intensity. Pain follows from slight shifts in the vertebral column, sometimes only a couple of millimeters, that occur with specific movements: arising from a low seat or standing from a low toilet are common provoking motions. The shift in the spine results, over ensuing hours, in profound muscle spasms and pain. Spine "listhesis" may reduce spontaneously, but in many cases spinal manipulation or repositioning maneuvers are required. Recognition of this syndrome is the key to diagnosis, referral to chiropractic or manual therapy may lead to ultra-rapid resolution.

Spinal stenosis is common in older adults. Pain may be widespread; ambulation is progressively limited. Comprehensive therapy potentially including surgery is necessary.

Nerve compression is discussed in Chapter 37; Coccydynia in Chapter 45.

Back pain emergencies are conditions potentially resulting in death or disability that present with back pain as a cardinal symptom, often identified clinically by the presence of one or more "red flags." Red flags is a term that describes critically important symptoms or signs associated with the potentially catastrophic causes of back pain. Red flags are considered effective in reducing unnecessary imaging of "benign" back pain. Red flags include fever, weakness, history of cancer, and other features, see Figure 36.1.

Despite the importance of utilizing imaging and other medical resources only when necessary, it is critically important to understand the role and value of the relevant imaging modalities (Fowler and Murinson 2015). Specifically, although MRIs are useful for identifying problems with soft tissues including spinal cord and nerves, they are expensive and a limited resource. For assessment of bone-based structures, X-ray is good for preliminary assessment, but for more detail or appraisal of suspected hemorrhage, CT remains the preferred modality. It is best to reserve MRI for patients with back pain when a potentially catastrophic back pain problem is suspected, or when back pain is severe and persistent (Figure 36.2).

Back pain emergencies include: vertebral fracture, epidural abscess, metastatic spinal cord compression, Guillain–Barre syndrome (sporadic postinfectious paralysis); described here (Figure 36.1).

Common and relevant conditions

Vertebral fracture can lead to spinal instability and spinal cord compression. This syndrome is less likely in younger patients with minimal trauma, but as people age, they become more prone to vertebral fracture with lesser degrees of trauma – due to decreases in both bone density and supporting muscle mass. Depending on the patient and the mechanics of injury, the nature of the fracture

will vary. Falls from height or at velocity can result in burst fracture, where the vertebral body essentially explodes under pressure. A fall from standing height can result in a wedge fracture, which when compromising only the anterior or posterior side of the spinal column, may not destabilize the column itself but can produce a bone fragment impinging on the spinal cord. A hairline fracture may be painful but not represent a serious risk to spinal stability or spinal cord integrity. The posterior elements of the vertebral bone, particularly the pedicles, can fracture when the vertebral body is displaced due to trauma. This may make the vertebral bone less stably positioned in the column, instability like this can result in both acute pain and a chronic syndrome of intermittent pain.

Epidural abscess is an infectious syndrome of the spinal column. It is usually associated with pain, often focal in nature, and neurological deficits which can be subtle at first but evolving to para- or quadriplegia, and incontinence. Fever may be present. The subtleness of symptoms means that vigilance in obtaining a credible neurological examination and documentation is important. The incidence of epidural abscess is relatively low, about 10 : 100000. It is more likely in patients with HIV, IVDA, alcoholism, diabetes, trauma, acupuncture, tattooing, and other immunocompromised states. The most common infectious agent is *Staphylococcus aureus*, and the patient most typically presenting with this condition is a 50-year-old male. Although abnormalities may be visible on CT, MRI is a more effective modality. An extended course of antibiotics is typical and drainage may be required.

Metastatic spinal cord compression is a common concomitant of cancer. Over half of cancer patients undergoing autopsy have spinal metastases, but only a fraction of these are symptomatic. Some cancers are more prone to spinal metastases, these include breast, lung, GI, prostate, and lymphoma. The classic

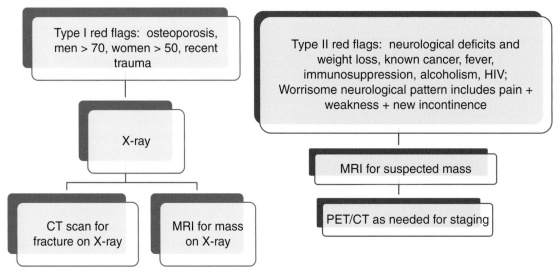

Figure 36.1 Comparison of Type I and Type II red flags for low back pain emergencies.

Pain Medicine at a Glance, First Edition. Beth B. Hogans.
© 2022 John Wiley & Sons Ltd. Published 2022 by John Wiley & Sons Ltd.

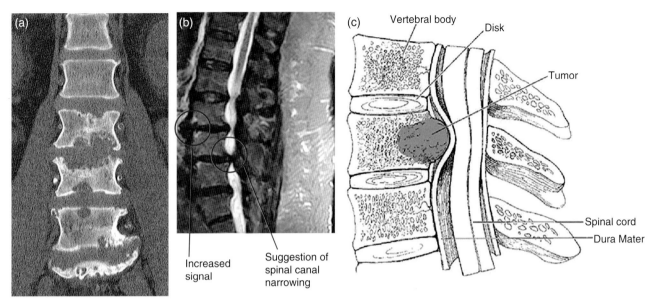

Figure 36.2 Imaging modalities and spinal abnormalities. (a) CT of lumbosacral spine with chronic changes. (b) MRI with acute findings and canal narrowing. (c) sketch illustrating epidural mass, metastatic replacement.

presentation is progressive pain, incontinence and weakness in the legs. While MRI is the preferred imaging modality, CT can be useful for assessing the stability of bones that have undergone metastatic invasion or replacement. Survival after metastatic spinal cord compression is poor. Treatment of spinal metastases can include NSAIDs, steroids, prescription pain medication, spinal orthotics, radiation (XRT), interventional and surgical approaches.

Other structural "red flag" back pain syndromes include **conus medullaris** syndrome, affecting the lower tip of the spinal cord and characterized by leg weakness with hyper-reflexia, bladder overactivity, and fecal incontinence; **cauda equina** syndrome, affecting the nerve roots below the level of the cord, potentially compressing roots asymmetrically and presenting with leg weakness with reduced reflexes, overflow incontinence of the bladder and decreased rectal tone; and **carcinomatous meningitis**, with metastatic dysfunction of multiple nerve roots in the lower spinal levels.

Guillain–Barre, in contrast to other back pain emergencies, does not require imaging. It can cause rapidly developing back pain that evolves into respiratory failure over the ensuing 24 hours.

The classic presentation is a patient who presents to the office with diffuse back pain and weakness progressing over the last 24 hours. Typically, the patient will not have elicitable reflexes, but early in the syndrome reflexes may be minimally present. The patient may or may not recall having had a recent viral infection e.g., URI or gastroenteritis, and may not yet have difficulty breathing. Because the risk of respiratory failure is so grave, immediate admission and treatment with IVIg or plasmapheresis is indicated for these patients.

Radiculopathy is a clinical urgency in many patients but is not technically a "red flag" emergency. It is a very common syndrome that affects millions of Americans each year. Associated with high levels of pain, 8/10 on average, radiculopathy reflects the compression of a spinal nerve root that may result in permanent weakness if not address promptly. For details, see Chapter 37.

Reference

Fowler, I. and Murinson, B. (2015). Spinal cord emergencies. DVCIPM assets.

Radiating pain in the lower extremity area most often arises from compression of lumbar or sacral nerve roots by spinal structures, e.g. radiculopathy with disc herniation; however, there are other causes of nerve compression, including sciatica due to piriformis syndrome, meralgia paresthetica, and tarsal tunnel syndrome; all addressed here.

Anatomy and innervation

There are three major mixed nerves that innervate the leg: the sciatic nerve posteriorly, and the femoral and obturator nerves anteriorly and medially; in addition, some sensory nerves, including the lateral femoral cutaneous nerve are involved in pain conditions. The femoral nerve extends into the saphenous nerve. The sciatic nerve divides into the tibial nerve, the peroneal (i.e. fibular) nerve, and the sural (pure sensory) nerve. These nerves are comprised of axons that arise from multiple lumbar and sacral nerve roots; compression of a nerve root at spine will produce a pain syndrome wherein shooting, aching, or severe pain will radiate into the leg, foot, or less often the groin area. The nerve roots exit the spine through "neural foramina."

Common and relevant conditions

Low lumbar and lumbosacral radiculopathy are the most common nerve compression syndromes representing over 70% of the radiculopathies among older adults, followed by cervical, and thoracic radiculopathies (Figure 37.1). Acute disc herniation per se is more common in early midlife because discs are still rubbery. Disc herniation typically follows overloaded twisting and lifting, jumping, or another precipitating event. In older adults, nerve compression occurs as a result of multifactorial compression: hypertrophied vertebral bones and facet joints, overgrowth of the upper and lower vertebral body surfaces, enlarged hypertrophied ligaments, and vertical distance decreases dramatically due to disc degeneration, altogether narrowing the cross-sectional area of neural foramina; obese patients can aggregate fat in the spinal spaces compressing nerve roots internally. Later in life, spinal stenosis ensues as degenerative changes accumulate. The challenge of nerve root compression is that nociceptive, inflammatory, and neuropathic pain forms, sensory deficits and motor weakness together can lead to permanent pain and disability (Murinson 2011). Although X-ray may show abnormalities, it is typically not sufficiently sensitive. Because fat, ligaments, discs, and soft tissues contribute to nerve compression, MRI is typically necessary to assess radicular symptoms.

The most common radicular syndromes are L4 (exiting between L4 and L5 vertebrae), L5 (sometimes referred to as L5-S1 due to exit point between L5 and S1 vertebrae), and S1 (exiting between S1 and S2) (Bähr and Frotscher 1998). The L4, L5, and S1 nerve root syndromes all present with pain that radiates below the knee, and these criteria, of radiation of pain to below the knee, was traditionally required for a diagnosis of "sciatica" or "lumbar" radiculopathy (Figure 37.2). Actually, sciatica can be caused by other nerve compression syndromes, e.g. piriformis syndrome, and lumbar radiculopathy doesn't always produce pain below the knee. Nonetheless, if weakness is a prominent symptom, and there is a clear operative lesion, such as a herniated, extruded or ruptured disc, surgery is associated with higher patient satisfaction and good outcomes. Radiculopathy due to less severe disc disruptions can resolve without surgery. Supportive care such as multimodal analgesia, activity modification, traction, manual therapy, ergonomics, can improve comfort and functional recovery. In some, interventional management is beneficial. Studies indicate that for patients with herniated discs not undergoing surgery, extended periods of time off work, e.g., seven weeks, are typical.

Atypical lumbar radiculopathies are (i) far less common and (ii) pain does not radiate below the knee. L3 radiculopathy radiates to the knee, L2 to the medial thigh, and L1 into the groin area. The weakness patterns reflect muscles innervated by the nerve roots, e.g., subtle quadriceps or obturator weakness (O'Brien 2010). These syndromes also arise from falls, lifting misadventures, or trauma.

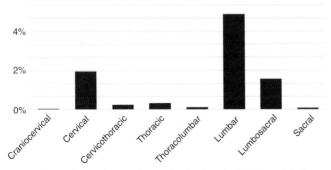

Figure 37.1 Diagnostic prevalence of radiculopathy in older adults by spinal level.

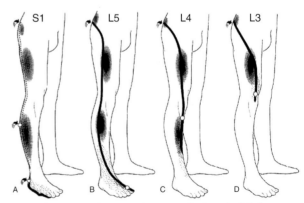

Figure 37.2 Patterns of common lumbar radicular pain, L3 (least common), L4, L5 (most common), S1. (Provenance uncertain).

Pain Medicine at a Glance, First Edition. Beth B. Hogans.
© 2022 John Wiley & Sons Ltd. Published 2022 by John Wiley & Sons Ltd.

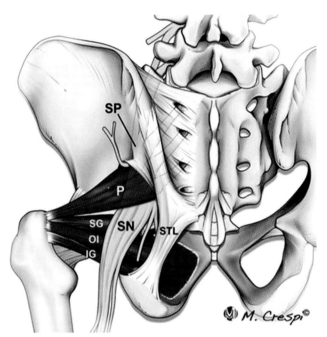

Figure 37.3 Illustration of sciatic nerve passes between piriformis and gemelli muscles deep in the buttock. Compression of the nerve by the muscles in spasm leads to a radiating sciatica-type pain condition, termed "piriformis syndrome." Source: Daniel Probst MD, et. al., (2019). © John Wiley & Sons.

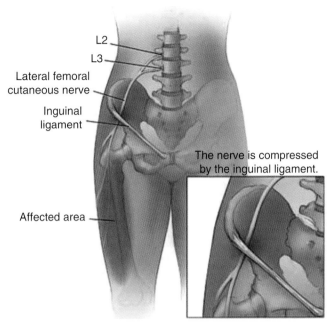

Figure 37.4 Illustration of meralgia paresthetica (MAYO – need substitute). Source: Used with permission of Mayo Foundation for Medical Education and Research, all rights reserved.

Piriformis syndrome-sciatica is a syndrome of pain radiating from buttock down into the leg and up toward the back. Often arising from motor vehicle rear-ending, traumatic falls, or similar trauma, damage to piriformis muscles, deep to gluteal muscles in the buttock, leads to persistent muscle spasms. The large sciatic nerve, running between the gemelli muscles, below, and the piriformis muscles "above," is compressed by these muscle spasms (Figure 37.3). The resulting syndrome partially resembles lumbosacral radiculopathy. Imagine the patient presenting with sciatica pain, who is then found not to have lumbosacral disc displacement – if the practitioner is not familiar with piriformis syndrome, the patient's experience of pain may be dismissed as "exaggerated," particular if litigation is pending. Piriformis muscle spasm can be appraised by physical therapist and knowledgeable front-line providers: for example, after warning the patient that you are going to palpate their gluteal area (bottom) with your hands, through their clothing, the provider will palpate deeply into the center of the buttock, with the gluteal muscles fully relaxed, it may be possible to perceive a firmness deep to the muscle, or patients will often exclaim that there is an area of painful tenderness, precisely in the location of the piriformis muscle. First line treatment involves specific daily stretching exercises, e.g. recumbent knee-to-chest stretches, and other physical therapy treatments.

Meralgia paresthetica produces neuropathic lateral thigh pain. Characterized by bothersome tingling, searing-burning, shooting, or aching pain in the lateral thigh, meralgia paresthetica is associated with obesity, pregnancy, or tight belt-wearing (Figure 37.4). The syndrome may be diagnosed with appropriate history, and physical exam findings of decreased sensation in the area of the lateral femoral cutaneous nerve, diagnostic utility of nerve conduction studies is limited. Treatment includes eliminating provoking compression where possible, and neuro-modulating agents such as gabapentin, as well as comprehensive pain management strategies.

References

Bähr, M. and Frotscher, M. (1998). Duus' Topical Diagnosis in Neurology: Anatomy, Physiology, Signs, Symptoms, 5. Thieme.

Murinson, B. (2011). Take Back Your Back: Everything You Need to Know to Effectively Reverse and Manage Back Pain. Beverly MA: Fair Winds Press.

O'Brien, M. (2010). Aids to the Examination of the Peripheral Nervous System 5. Saunders.

Knee pain is the most prevalent cause of chronic pain worldwide. Vying with back pain for limiting mobility and diminishing quality of life, knee dysfunction prevents instrumental activities of daily living like cleaning, shopping, and preparing meals. Acute knee pain is prevalent across age groups whereas chronic knee pain is very prevalent in older patients and presents future challenges as people live longer and have conditions that interfere with safe NSAID administration (Gage et al. 2012). Knee OA has lifetime prevalence of 45%, rising to 60% for the obese (Neogi 2013).

Anatomy and innervation

The knee is a synovial joint between the distal femur, proximal tibial, the patella sits anteriorly. It is bound medially and laterally by medial and lateral collateral ligaments (MCL and LCL) and stabilized internally with anterior and posterior cruciate ligaments (ACL and PCL) (Figure 38.1). Muscular support from quadriceps, hamstrings, and sartorius muscles helps to prevent injury. Internal joint systems of shock absorption include synovial fluid and cartilaginous semilunate meniscuses located medially and laterally (Figure 38.2).

The knee is innervated by branches of femoral, obturator, peroneal, and tibial nerves. Femoral supplies proximal anterior knee, obturator the medial knee, tibial the postero-medial knee with a branch to distal knee medially, and peroneal the posterior knee laterally with an anterior branch anterior to the lateral distal knee. The peroneal nerve is vulnerable to compression at the fibular head, this may lead to motor dysfunction, i.e. foot drop, as well as a painful neuropathy. Knowledge of knee innervation, most

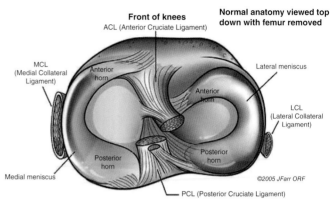

Figure 38.2 Interior view of the knee from above with femur remove, illustrating relationship of meniscuses, and ligaments. This is the right knee. Source: © 2005, JFarr ORF.

important for nerve blocks, may inform primary care when topical agents such as lidocaine are considered.

Clinical assessment

For acute knee pain, assess localization to medial or lateral knee – each prone to different injuries. Inciting factors for pain are critically important in diagnosis: runners are prone to patellar-femoral syndrome (anterior distal knee pain), dancers are prone to meniscus injury (lateral or medial pain). On exam, assess passive and active range of motion, weight-bearing, effusion, surface temperature, tenderness to palpation, and provocative maneuvers.

Basics of treatment

Acute pain in the knee begins on standard treatment according to the RICE-M protocol. Immediate attention to Resting the knee, Ice (cold compress), Compression and support to the knee, Elevation when possible, and Medication appropriate for pain and inflammation are essential (Finlayson 2014). Exam findings determine whether diagnostic imaging is needed: MRI is not needed acutely for most knee injury, but X-ray may be useful to exclude dislocation, fracture, arthritis, or malignancy. Treatment proceeds according to type of injury (Figure 38.3). Bracing provides comfort, reduces pain, and supports movement during the early-phase recovery, sustained use requires orthopedic consultation.

Chronic knee pain treatment may vary depending on the causes of pain and the severity of knee degeneration. Strengthening is a first-line element of management in many types of chronic knee pain. PT and home exercise are essential.

Ergonomics are indispensable for long-term management of chronic knee pain. Careful attention to foot, ankle, and leg positioning with gait may be gauged by the primary care practitioner with a simple

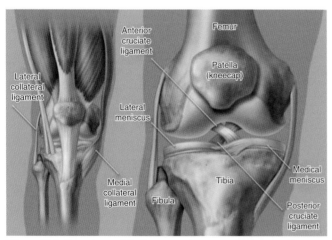

Figure 38.1 Two views of the knee, anterior anatomical view with muscles, medial, and lateral collateral ligaments; view with muscles, nerves, and tendons removed – bones, meniscuses, and ligaments are visible. This is the right knee.

Pain Medicine at a Glance, First Edition. Beth B. Hogans.
© 2022 John Wiley & Sons Ltd. Published 2022 by John Wiley & Sons Ltd.

Activity	Provoking movement	Injury	Exam notes and pain features
Field sports, court sports	Knee hyperextension; stepping with turn	ACL	Anterior translation of tibia with Lachman maneuver
Field sports	Fall onto flexed knee	PCL	Posterior drawer
Martial arts, field sports	Blow to the lateral knee	MCL	**Pain with strain on medial knee** (valgus strain (lateral knee pressure))
Running, cycling	Repeated movement	Iliotibial band	More common than LCL, **sharp pain in proximal lateral knee with motion**
Running	Repeated pounding gait	Patellofemoral syndrome	Negative exam, **diffuse distal knee pain (below patella)**
Dancing, field sports, skiing	Twisting with planted foot	Meniscus	**Tender to palpation along joint line**, decreased ROM

Figure 38.3 Common knee injuries with provoking activities and examination notes.

walking test. Any deviation from normal merits evaluation by a gait specialist. Some practitioners send patients to the local running store, this may serve the pragmatic purpose of cost-effective improvements in gait when local practice patterns push patients toward expensive custom orthotics. Nonetheless, some podiatrists will provide less expensive orthotic options like lifts.

Anti-inflammatory medications are part of many treatment regimens. Before treating carefully assess co-morbid conditions. Patients with conditions such as GERD cannot take NSAIDs routinely. Patients at risk for heart disease and stroke, as well as those with risk factors for vascular disease need to limit NSAID exposure to the minimum necessary. Renal dysfunction precludes use. With aging, more patients are unable to tolerate NSAID treatment.

Topical agents are often used in the treatment of chronic knee pain. The nerves supplying the knee joint are relatively superficial in non-obese patients and the knee is easily accessed for treatment application. Capsaicin topically must be applied four to five times daily for efficacy. Topical lidocaine and topical NSAIDS, e.g. voltaren and Pennsaid are also used. Counterirritants (Biofreeze, Bengay) are available over the counter.

Self-management is key in patients with knee pain and includes: warming the knee with a heating pad, cooling the knee – especially after exercise or strain, activity modification, attention to body mechanics, moderate daily exercise, and proper stretching.

Weight loss is indispensable in chronic knee pain. Each pound lost provides extra relief to the knee. Engage patients using motivational interviewing to identify realistic goals, and healthier lifestyle choices.

Interventional management of knee pain involves the injection of steroids or viscous solutions into the knee (Gregory and Martin 2017). Steroids are often coinjected with a local anesthetic so there may be immediate relief in the first hours after the procedure followed by a transient return of pain followed by some weeks of pain relief. Repeated steroid injections have been associated with systemic effects of diabetes, osteoporosis, and serious infections. Viscous solutions based on hyaluronic acid derivatives can be injected (Syn-visc) providing additional fluid cushioning with relief for several months at a time.

Joint replacement is reserved for advanced knee degeneration not amenable to other modalities, nonetheless 700 000 knee replacements occur annually in the U.S. (Kurtz et al. 2007). Knee replacement requires a commitment on the part of patient to engage actively in rehabilitation. Patients are often surprised by how difficult it is to get the knee range of motion back after surgery. Anticipatory physical therapy, or "pre-hab" before surgery yields improved outcomes.

References

Finlayson, C. (2014). Knee injuries in the young athlete. Pediatric Annals 43 (12): e282–e290.

Gage, B.E., NM, M.I., Collins, C.L. et al. (2012). Epidemiology of 6.6 million knee injuries presenting to United States emergency departments from 1999 through 2008. Academic Emergency Medicine 19 (4): 378–385.

Gregory, M and Martin, M.D. (2017). Patient education: total knee replacement (arthroplasty) (beyond the basics). https://www.uptodate.com/contents/total-knee-replacement-arthroplasty-beyond-the-basics (accessed 27 September 2017).

Kurtz, S., Ong, K., Lau, E. et al. (2007). Projections of primary and revision hip and knee arthroplasty in the United States from 2005 to 2030. The Journal of Bone and Joint Surgery. American Volume 89: 780.

Neogi, T. (2013). The epidemiology and impact of pain in osteoarthritis. Osteoarthritis and Cartilage 21 (9): 1145–1153.

Foot and ankle pain is associated with worse long-term health outcomes. For example, a young person with an ankle sprain is more likely to develop obesity. Foot and ankle injuries are highly prevalent in the younger population, peaking in the late teens and decreasing steadily with age. Ankle sprains account for more emergency room encounters than any other injury to the lower extremity (Lambers et al. 2012) and can lead to a chronic cycle of ankle instability, pain, and arthritis, Table 39.1.

Table 39.1 Incidence of sprains of the lower quarter.

Site	Annual incidence per 100 000 (Lambers et al. 2012)
Ankle	206
Hip, pelvis, and lumbar spine	155
Knee	102
Foot and toe	46

Anatomy and physiology

Comprised of a synovial joint located where the distal tibia and fibula meet to form a downward facing arch over the dome of the talus, the true ankle joint allows hinge-motion. The talus sits atop the calcaneus connected by multiple ligaments and synovial capsule. Anterior are the navicular and cuneiform bones, which connect anteriorly to the metatarsal and thence to the tarsal bones of the toes. The bones of the foot form medial and lateral longitudinal arches, and an anterior transverse arch is present normally as well. The bones of the foot, supported by ligaments, give rise to the flexibility, stability, and adaptability of the human foot (Figure 39.1).

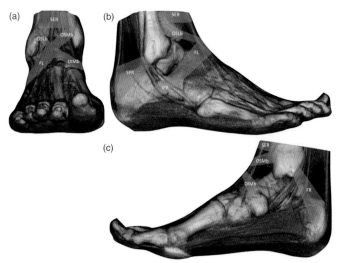

Figure 39.1 Bones and ligaments of the foot and ankle, with (a) anterior, (b) lateral and (c) medial views.

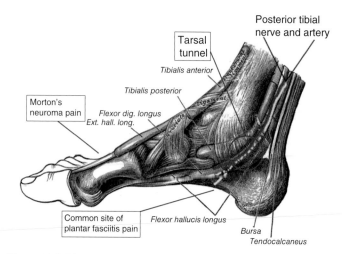

Figure 39.2 Diagram illustrating selected common foot ailments. Kiel J (2020)/StatPearls Publishing LLC/CC BY 4.0.

Branches of the peroneal and saphenous (from femoral) nerves innervate the foot dorsally, the sural nerve laterally, and the tibial nerve inferiorly (plantar surface). The tibial nerve traverses the posterior calf, passes behind the medial malleolus and enters the tarsal tunnel, Figure 39.2. The peroneal nerve is split into deep and superficial branches supplying distal and proximal dorsal foot. The sural nerve is frequently studied in nerve conduction studies (assessing generalized or diffuse neuropathies). Vascular supply to the foot is often compromised in patients with diabetes and advanced peripheral vascular disease, in addition the foot can be subject to venous stasis.

Clinical assessment

In evaluating an episode of acute foot and ankle pain in primary practice, it is most important to consider the potential etiology of the problem. Evaluation of the ankle for range of motion, edema, tenderness, weight-bearing, and strength is essential; and circulation, edema, coloration, atrophic changes, tenderness to palpation, and provocative maneuvers also included. The foot is prone to traumatic penetration, blisters, abrasions, inflammatory responses, or infectious processes, which can develop and worsen rapidly. Test ankle reflexes and proprioception, and if neuropathy is suspected, sensitivity to sharp stimuli should be assessed with careful attention to either diminished or heightened pain sensation.

Basics of treatment

Acute pain in the ankle and foot follows the RICE-M protocol, and diagnostic imaging and bracing steps of Chapter 38.

Pain Medicine at a Glance, First Edition. Beth B. Hogans.
© 2022 John Wiley & Sons Ltd. Published 2022 by John Wiley & Sons Ltd.

Table 39.2 Distinguishing features of pain syndromes in the foot and ankle.

Location of pain and quality	Provoking activity	Injury	Exam features	Treatment notes
Aching pain over medial ball of foot	Improper foot wear, excessive high-heel wearing	Bunion	Boney deformity with valgus of hallux	Proper footwear, medication, injection, or surgical revision
Pain with tight shoes or lateral foot compression	Chronic ill-fitting shoes	Morton's neuroma	Pressing between fourth & fifth metatarsal bones provokes pain	Proper footwear, medication, injection, or excision
Sharp pain in sole of foot upon first step in morning	Putting weight on feet, gaining weight, new shoes, excessive standing	Plantar fasciitis	Palpation of sole near heel may provoke pain	Heel wedge, stretching exercises for gastrocnemius and plantar fascia, ice massage
Burning pain first in toes then migrating proximally	Worse at night, worse after daytime activity	Diffuse small fiber neuropathy	Foot appears normal or may have atrophic changes or purpura	Gabapentinoid, evaluate for diabetes/other causes, ensure proper footwear

Chronic foot and ankle pain treatment may vary depending on the causes of pain and the suspected cause. Several specifics of treatment are noted in Table 39.2.

Careful attention to foot, ankle, and leg positioning with gait may be gauged by the primary care practitioner with the "observed walking" test (Goldman 2016). Any deviation from normal merits evaluation by a gait specialist such as a podiatrist.

Before medicating foot pain, consider whether the pain is inflammatory, nociceptive, or neuropathic. NSAIDs may help with inflammatory or nociceptive pain, but caution is appropriate (see Chapter 38). NSAIDs and acetaminophen do not relieve neuropathic pain; indeed, patients with no relief from NSAIDs or acetaminophen may have neuropathic pain.

Topical agents can alleviate foot and ankle pain. Capsaicin can provoke severe burning in neuropathic pain and should be avoided. Topical lidocaine can help with peripheral neuropathy pain but can only be applied once daily. Some patients like the convenience of lidocaine patches, which can be cut to fit the problematic area. Topical NSAIDS (Voltaren and Pennsaid) and counterirritants (Biofreeze, Bengay) may alleviate arthritic conditions but not neuropathy.

Self-management is very important in patients with foot and ankle pain: warming with a heating pad, cooling with cold-pack application – especially after exercise, and activity modification with attention to body mechanics, modified exercise, bracing, orthotics, and proper stretching. Those with neuropathy will report worse pain when the feet are warmed. Open, but supportive and protective footwear may provide substantive relief. Weight loss is important to the long-term management of chronic ankle and foot pain.

Interventional management of foot and ankle pain can involve the injection of steroids. Surgical management is reserved for advanced degeneration not amenable to other modalities.

Plantar fasciitis is an acute inflammatory foot condition that may present as an abrupt first episode of alarmingly severe posterior arch pain in someone who is otherwise very healthy, Figure 39.2. Heel lifts may help. Proper recognition and management can prevent the condition from becoming a chronic hindrance.

Tarsal tunnel syndrome is the lower limb equivalent of carpal tunnel, Figure 39.2. The syndrome can result in pain radiating into the foot arch or into the medial ankle. Biomechanical, e.g. ankle position, footwear, excessive use; and systemic factors, e.g. diabetes may contribute to the syndrome (Kiel 2020). Diagnosis can be made with detailed neurological exam and confirmed with nerve condition studies or response to podiatric treatment trials.

Morton's neuroma is (nonmalignant) nerve injury and sensitivity to compression with foot pain provoked by pressure on the forefoot. The small nerves that travel between the third and fourth tarsal bones in the forefoot are damaged. To test for these, press on the forefoot from above and below, over the inter-tarsal spaces, when a neuroma is present, the patient will note pain. Lateral forefoot pressure (squeeze from sides) also provokes pain. Neuromas may be detected by ultrasound (although this does not typically need to precede referral) and can be treated by podiatrists; gabapentinoids may reduce pain.

Foot and ankle pain syndromes include nociceptive, inflammatory, neuropathic, and combined-mechanism pain syndromes. Treatment is important for ambulation and to reduce the negative impacts on overall health.

References

Goldman, S. (2016). *Walking Well Again*. Baltimore, MD: Facilitation Press, LLC.

Kiel J. Tarsal tunnel syndrome. In: *StatPearls*. Kaiser K. Treasure Island, FL: Stat Pearls Publishing; 2020. https://www.ncbi.nlm.nih.gov/books/NBK513273/ (accessed 22 June 2020).

Lambers, K., Ootes, D., and Ring, D. (2012). Incidence of patients with lower extremity injuries presenting to US emergency departments by anatomic region, disease category, and age. *Clinical Orthopaedics and Related Research* 470: 284–290.

Headache emergencies are prevalent in clinical practice and are especially relevant for primary care, ER providers, and neurologists. Headache is, at the core, a subjective phenomenon, but in headache emergencies, the objective features strongly shape the differential diagnosis (Table 40.1). For example, when evaluating an acute headache, it is very important to know if the headache is associated with a rash, as in meningococcal meningitis; acute focal neurological deficits; fever, as in infectious processes of meningitis or encephalitis; or visual loss, characteristic of temporal arteritis (Table 40.2).

Table 40.1 Typical temporal course and major exam findings of major headache emergencies.

Common headache emergencies	Timing	General findings	Neurological
Subarachnoid hemorrhage	Thunderclap headache, onset over seconds	HBP	Transient loss of consciousness Followed by lucid interval Followed by depressed mental status
Meningitis	Hyper-acute, worsening over minutes-to-hours	Fever Neck stiffness Rash (meningococc.)	Headache Other findings may be mild Seizure and focal deficits may exist
Encephalitis	Acute/subacute, worsens over hours-to-days	Fever	Focal deficits, e.g. seizure Depressed consciousness
Temporal arteritis	Subacute with potential for stepwise worsening	Weight loss Fever	Jaw claudication, shoulder/hip pain Visual loss progressing to blindness

Table 40.2 Highlights of testing, imaging, and clinical notes for major headache emergencies.

Common headache emergencies	Test results	Imaging	Clinical notes
Subarachnoid hemorrhage	Cerebrospinal fluid (CSF): elevated RBCs	CT is part of search for subarachnoid blood, may image for aneurysm also	Intensive care management, risk for re-bleeding
Meningitis	CSF: markedly elevated WBCs, may have neutrophilic predominance	Per protocol, should not delay therapy; needed if focal neuro-deficits	Antibiotics without delay, minutes matter as this can be rapidly fatal
Encephalitis	CSF: elevated WBCs, may mostly lymphocytes	Per protocol, should not delay therapy; needed if focal neuro-deficits	Antiviral agents, send CSF for virologic testing, empiric treatment protocol
Temporal arteritis[a]	Elevated ESR (sedimentation rate)	Not typically performed; arterial biopsy needed - shows vasculitis	Urgent ophthalmologic referral for assessment and TA biopsy, steroids

[a] May have insidious onset.

Lumbar puncture (LP) is often an essential element of evaluating headache emergencies, but in patients with focal neurological deficits consider whether to image before LP, potentially to ensure that no space occupying lesion is present (Bähr and Frotscher 1998; Ropper et al. 2014, Figure 40.1). Due to the rapid and destructive nature of brain infections, in the case that diagnostic testing might delay treatment, rapid initiation of empiric treatment typically proceeds.

Subarachnoid hemorrhage (SAH) is a headache emergency. The risk of fatality is high in unrecognized SAH. A thunderclap headache with a transient lucid interval followed by progressive decline in alertness, i.e., altered mental status, is considered classic but not universal. The diagnostic tests include CT and LP for red

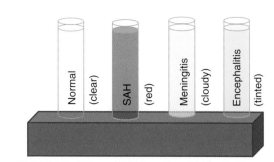

Figure 40.1 Classic CSF appearance, varies with diagnosis, may visualize at bedside and appearance will be noted in lab report.

Pain Medicine at a Glance, First Edition. Beth B. Hogans.
© 2022 John Wiley & Sons Ltd. Published 2022 by John Wiley & Sons Ltd.

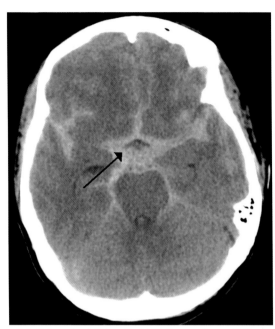

Figure 40.2 Subarachnoid blood in SAH. Source: James Heilman, MD/ Wikimedia Commons. CC BY-SA 3.0

blood cells in the cerebrospinal fluid (CSF) (Figure 40.2). The diagnostic utility of CT for blood is high and preferred to MRI. These patients require hospital management, often in intensive care. Evaluation for aneurysms is critical to ascertaining the source of bleeding, and neurosurgical involvement is usually appropriate.

Meningitis is another headache emergency. The diagnosis of meningitis is highly time-sensitive, and death will result if treatment is not started immediately. In the event that it is not possible to perform an LP, antibiotics must be started with broad-spectrum coverage until diagnostic test results are available. Because the meninges cover the brain and the infection does not directly disable specific brain centers, the presence of focal neurological deficits has traditionally been viewed as less likely, although seizure and depressed consciousness can result. The classic presentation of acute bacterial meningitis is severe headache, stiff neck, and fever. This is an acute illness. The neck is stiff primarily in flexion as this is a result of nocifensive (protective) anti-flexion in order to prevent tension of the brain and by extension, spinal meninges. Meningococcal meningitis evolves very rapidly, over hours, to coma and is accompanied by a petechial rash in 50%. Immediate institution of therapy is paramount. The common meningitis of infancy and early childhood has been virtually eliminated by vaccination. Pneumococccal meningitis is observed in those with recent lung, ear, or sinus infections, as well as the elderly and those with alcohol use disorder. Staphylococcal infections arise in those with shunts or instrumentation. Listeria may occur in the elderly. Demographic information is important to anticipating the likely pathogen and planning antibiotic coverage. Hospitalization with intensive care as needed, prolonged administration of antibiotics, and specialist involvement is typical.

Encephalitis is often viral in etiology and may be associated with focal neurological findings. The classic triad of headache, fever, and focal neurological signs, including seizure, should raise concerns for encephalitis, although brain abscess can present similarly. Neuroimaging, CT generally, should precede LP to evaluate the CSF. White cell counts in CSF are elevated but lower than in bacterial meningitis, with lymphocytic predominance characteristic. Herpes simplex encephalitis (HSE) is the most common cause of sporadic encephalitis and should be treated with an appropriate antiviral regimen. In many cases, antiviral therapy is started immediately pending test results. The administration of antiviral agents is essential and time-sensitive in HSE as the pathogen produces a fulminant hemorrhagic destruction of the affected cortex, which results in permanent loss of associated neurological function.

Temporal arteritis is distinctive in the headache emergencies in that onset is insidious, but patients may present with acute headache and visual loss. The visual loss may be intermittent at first but rapidly progresses to permanent blindness. Temporal arteritis is a systemic condition of older adults with prodromal symptoms, including weight loss, proximal joint pains, and fatigue. Key features of claudication with chewing, headache, and visual loss prompt patients to seek medical attention. Although "classic," palpable, tender temporal arteries are not always present. The most essential initial diagnostic test is Erythrocyte Sedimentation Rate (ESR). This will be marked elevated in most patients with temporal arteritis. Referral to ophthalmology for urgent evaluation and temporal artery biopsy is appropriate, but steroids may be started immediately if the diagnosis is likely.

Other life-limiting causes of acute headache include hypertensive encephalopathy, hemorrhagic stroke, brain abscess, vasculitis, cerebral vasospasm, and brain tumor. Vital signs, neuro-imaging, and basic lab testing will demonstrate the process involved in most of these with the exception of CNS vasculitis and vasospastic syndromes, which will require vascular imaging. In some cases, more invasive testing is needed to diagnose acute headache syndromes.

Benign, severe headache can cause patients to present for acute care for evaluation and management. Once immediate neuroimaging, typically CT, is completed and the ER team is satisfied that the life-threatening causes of headache have been appropriately excluded, treatment can turn to protocols for pain and symptom management.

Patients with migraine often experience very severe throbbing hemicranial pain. For someone with a first migraine, this may feel like "the worst headache of their lives" and be accompanied by photophobia, nausea, and vomiting. Headache protocols are widely used by hospitals to address the pain and associated symptoms of acute benign headache.

References

Bähr, M. and Frotscher, M. (1998). *Duus' Topical Diagnosis in Neurology: Anatomy, Physiology, Signs, Symptoms*, 5e. Stuttgart: Thieme.

Puyó, D. (2013). Subarachnoid hemorrhage. https://radiopaedia.org/cases/subarachnoid-haemorrhage-4 (accessed 8 February 2020).

Ropper, A.H., Samuels, M.A., and Klein, J. (2014). *Adams and Victor's Principles of Neurology*, 10e. New York, NY: McGraw-Hill Education.

Headaches have lifetime prevalence of 90% and affect 50% of adults annually (IASP Headache Factsheet 2017). Tension type headaches represent the most prevalent form of headache – about 50% of headaches. Migraine headaches are experienced by about 20% of adults with a female preponderance and genetic predisposition. Because migraine is so severe compared with more moderate tension headaches, it is the main headache seen in clinical encounters. It is important to distinguish so-called "benign" syndromic headaches from more ominous headaches which may be secondary to other disease processes. For this reason, physical exam is a mainstay of headache assessment. Diagnostic testing may include neuroimaging for patients with focal abnormalities, serum or blood testing when headaches secondary to infections or inflammatory illness is suspected, and lumbar puncture in selected settings. So-called "benign" headaches can have a devastating impact on a person's productivity and quality of life. Although subjective, headaches have profound, observable effects on patients, families, and providers. Adopting a systematic approach to headache assessment and management, one which allows patients to feel supported and understood while building a healthy therapeutic alliance are cornerstone concepts of pain medicine that are especially relevant in patients with disabling acute or chronic headache.

Basic evaluation

Begin with a description of the cardinal features of the pain: quality, region, severity, timing, usually-associated symptoms, alleviating, and worsening factors. Some patients will have more than one headache type. It is important to help the patient distinguish these headaches to tailor treatment for each type. A **headache calendar** is a useful tool for communicating with patients about their headaches (Figures 41.1). The patient completes the calendar each day, rating the intensity of headache pain experienced using a numerical scale (0–10). The patient brings this calendar with them to appointments and this organizes the discussion about headache severity, frequency, plans for and response to treatment. Patients with multiple headache types can enter codes to indicate which headache is experienced, e.g. (i) left temporal pounding-throbbing, (ii) whole head squeezing, (iii): aura without headache."

Physical examination should include appraisal of neurological function. A structured neurological exam is appropriate prior to imaging, either performed by the PCP or an experienced specialist. The American Academy of Neurology recommends neuroimaging, i.e. MRI only for those patients with neurological deficits. Neurological examination for headache is described in Appendix 1. Musculoskeletal exam of head, neck, and shoulders can reveal treatable headache forms, e.g. cervicogenic headache.

Tension type headache

The classic tension type headache (TTH) is a bifrontal pressure-like band around the head that is moderately severe and worsening over the day (Mayo Clinic 2021). The associated symptoms may include neck and shoulder pain, occipital pain, but not nausea, vomiting, aura, or photophobia. Allodynia or tenderness of soft tissues to palpation may be present over the head, neck, and shoulders but not prominent. When severe, the pain of TTH may radiate to the vertex or top of the head. Poor sleep can both trigger tension-type headache, and predispose to chronic tension-type headache (Rains et al. 2015). Tension type headache is associated with decreased quality of life and comorbid depression makes the effects of tension type headache more profound. Pathophysiology is poorly understood, but most of these respond to standard over-the-counter analgesia. The most pressing challenge in TTH is those patients who are at risk for frequent, intractable, or chronic headache. In some patients with frequent TTH, a syndrome of chronic daily headache or medication overuse headache can

Sunday	Monday	Tuesday	Wednesday	Thursday	Friday	Saturday
Type: A Intensity: 8 Duration: 2 h Start: late AM			Type: B Intensity: 5 Duration: 4 h Start: PM			
Type: A Intensity: 8 Duration: 2 h Start: late AM		Type: C Intensity: 6 Duration: 1 h Start: AM				
Legend: A type headache – throbbing half-headed; B type – band-like pressure; C type – pressure over left sinus						

Figure 41.1 Headache calendars are essential for gathering sufficiently detailed data in order to make decision-making possible for patient and provider. The legend is defined by the patient according to their headaches.

Pain Medicine at a Glance, First Edition. Beth B. Hogans.
© 2022 John Wiley & Sons Ltd. Published 2022 by John Wiley & Sons Ltd.

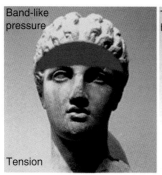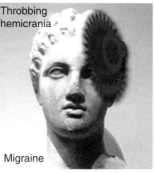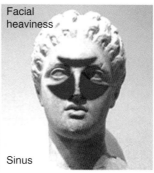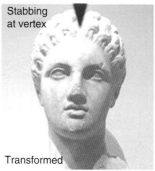

Figure 41.2 Headaches are principally subjective; patient-reported features lead to classification. Selected common headaches are depicted here, e.g. tension – band-like pressure, migraine – throbbing hemicrania, etc. The figure here is an ancient marble sculpture of a goddess, potentially Hygeia, daughter of Asklepios, the Greek god of medicine (The Metropolitan Museum of Art 2020). Source: Rogers Fund, 1910. Public Domain

develop, especially in patients taking daily acetaminophen. One strategy can be to alternate acetaminophen with NSAID. For chronic TTH, see Chapter 42.

Migraine headache

Migraine headache is chiefly characterized by severely painful throbbing hemicrania associated with photo- and phonophobia and often with nausea or vomiting. Migraines are highly prevalent, affecting about 20% of women and a smaller percentage of men, with a female:male ratio of 2–3:1. Migraines have substantive heritability of about 0.3. Migraines are complex polygenic disorders that may be autosomal dominant. Mitochondrial mechanisms have been implicated by some, and rare mitochondrial variant migraines are known (Yorns 2013). Vascular reactivity and inflammatory mediators, especially calcitonin gene-related product (CGRP) are implicated. New therapies including anti-CGRP antibodies are now FDA approved. Nonetheless, rapid administration of NSAIDs or triptans remains a central tenant of treatment for most patients.

Treatment of migraines is a collaborative endeavor for any but the most basic migraine. For simple migraine, avoidance of triggers, regular meals, appropriate hydration, and ready access to OTC analgesia are often the most effective measures.

Dietary supplement regimens are popular with patients and most of these endeavors to improve energy metabolism. Favored agents include riboflavin, CoQ 10, Alphalipoic acid, magnesium, niacin, and carnitine.

Occipital neuralgia

Occipital neuralgia stems from irritation or compression of the greater occipital nerve which innervates the posterior head. It can be worse in persons with chronic neck strain or extension. Injections

are popular for management but treatment of musculoskeletal concomitants may be helpful.

Secondary headache

Headache can arise for a variety of causes some of which are quite ominous. Brain tumor can present with insidiously worsening headache; typically accompanied by neurological deficits which precipitate neuroimaging, the prognosis is highly variable and tumors can range from benign meningiomas to aggressive glioblastoma multiforme. Inflammatory and autoimmune disorders such as sarcoid, Lyme disease, vasculitis, brain abscess, and lupus can present with headache. Sinusitis can present with headache, the hallmark characteristic being headache that worsens with leaning forward. Sleep apnea may present with headache, daily headache on awakening generally requires careful consideration of diagnostic testing.

References

IASP Headache Factsheet (2017). https://www.iasp-pain.org/files/Content/ContentFolders/GlobalYearAgainstPain2/HeadacheFactSheets/1-Epidemiology.pdf (accessed 21 June 2017).

Mayo Clinic (2021). Tension Headache. http://www.mayoclinic.org/diseases-conditions/tension-headache/home/ovc-20211413 (accessed 2 January 2021).

Rains, J.C., Davis, R.E., and Smitherman, T.A. (2015). Tension-type headache and sleep. Current Neurology and Neuroscience Reports 15 (2): 520.

The Metropolitan Museum of Art (2020). Marble head of a goddess, 4th century B.C. https://www.metmuseum.org/art/collection/search/248268 (accessed 2 August 2020).

Yorns, W.R. (2013). Mitochondrial dysfunction in migraine. Seminars in Pediatric Neurology 20 (3): 188–193.

General features and diagnostic guidance

Chronic headaches affect patients multiple times a month for months on end, specific definitions vary but typically this includes 15 headache days per month over a period of at least three months. Some chronic headaches have specific temporal criteria. The most reliable reference for these details is the **International Classification of Headache Disorders.** This resource defines criteria for essentially all recognized headache disorders making headache definition transparent and uniform. Available without charge online, it should be consulted liberally. Because correct diagnosis leads to correct treatment: Utilize reliable resources and apply definitions carefully.

Before refining diagnosis, first tease apart multitype headaches. Although this could seem too complex for primary practice, one technique is to explain to the patient that there might be multiple types, discuss with the patient how they might recognize these and propose a coding system to combine with ordinary headache calendar-keeping (please see Figure 41.1). Give the patient permission to define their own system as this can increase engagement, then schedule a follow-up appointment in about four weeks. Offer some safe nonopioid treatment options but let the patient know that it will take time to work together and resolve the headaches. At the next visit, review the headache calendar together and discuss potential patterns. Find a headache that seems recognizable and begin pharmacological treatment for that headache, together with the patient commit to some safe nonpharmacological pain management therapies. Work to identify headache triggers, and recognize perpetuating behaviors and comorbid conditions: overmedication, smoking, sleep apnea; address these directly or through referral. Sleep apnea affects >25% of adult males and 10% of females, increases with age and often presents with chronic headache. The STOP-BANG screening instrument is a rapidly administered tool that appraises risks for sleep apnea (Chung et al. 2008; Klinger et al. 2018).

Systematically caring about, carefully guiding, and confidently inspiring patients to anticipate positive results from treatment can have a beneficial effect as powerful as some medications [Colloca]. If you are concerned that this "placebo/expectancy" effect will diminish over time, you can expect that the benefits of comprehensive management will strengthen over time and the patient will improve. Headaches are incredibly common and headache competency in primary practice is a simple, deeply compassionate act as the waiting times for many specialty headache clinics are many months.

It is absolutely essential to use the multimodal treatment plan graphic in counseling the patient. Use it to plan treatment; give a copy to the patient, explore options, work patiently and without becoming discouraged – the graphic itself can inspire hope for

Comprehensive headache treatment: examples

Psychological support
Cognitive behavioral therapy
Mindfulness-based stress reduction
Acceptance-commitment therapy
Substance cessation

Ergonomic adaptation
Avoidance of triggers
Regular eating and sleeping
Consistent hydration
Spine/neck support

Mind–body
Gentle or seated yoga
Chi-gong
Acupuncture/acupressure
Trigger points: neck, head, shoulders

Physical activity
Moderate daily exercise
Neck strengthening
Stretching and posture

PAIN

Sleep
Sleep hygiene practices
Neck and head support

Passive strategies
(below the line)

'Safe standards'
Intermittent (avoid daily use)
Acetaminophen
NSAIDs

Pain modulation
Pain-active anticonvulsants,
e.g. topiramate
Pain-active antidepressants

**Interventions
(in reserve)**
Occipital nerve block
Botox injections

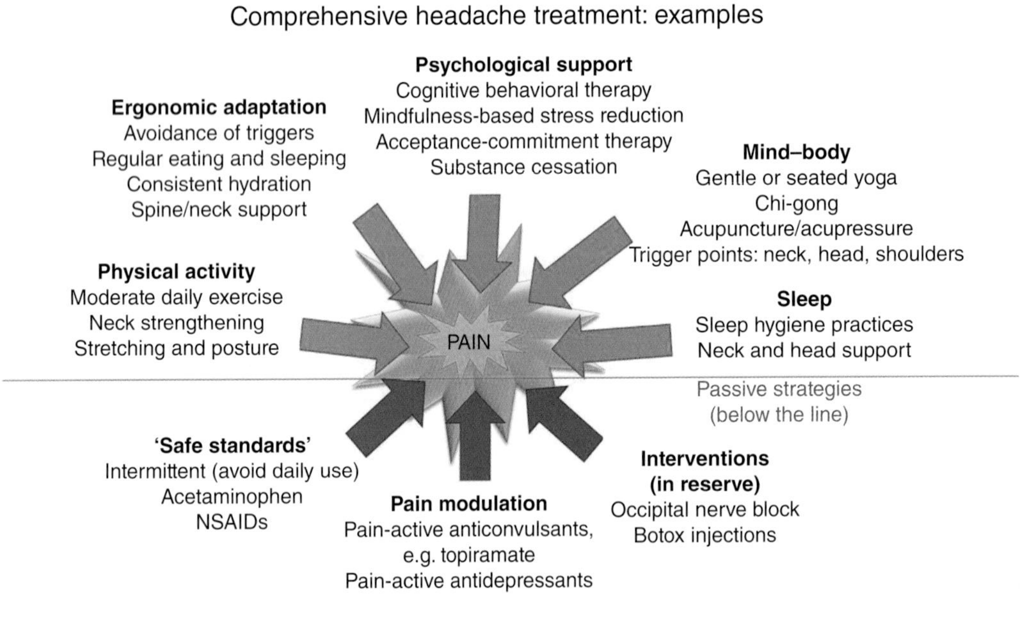

Figure 42.1 Comprehensive pain management is highly effective for chronic headache. Share and discuss this approach with your patients.

effective treatments in patients (Figure 42.1). One of the remarkable things about headache is how much headache can hurt and how completely disabling it is, without evidence of damage to the brain. This point can be discussed, at an appropriate moment, to offer reassurance.

Common and relevant conditions

Chronic tension headache is a frequent, persistent headache evolving from an episodic tension-type headache, lasting longer than three months (International Classification of Headache

Pain Medicine at a Glance, First Edition. Beth B. Hogans.
© 2022 John Wiley & Sons Ltd. Published 2022 by John Wiley & Sons Ltd.

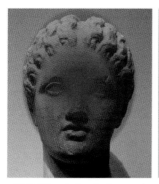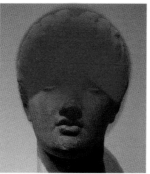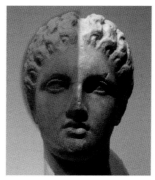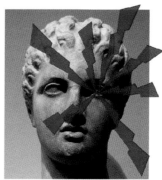

Figure 42.2 Chronic headaches can be very impairing: perturbing focus or in some cases all meaningful function. Patterns include whole head, vertex-overwhelming, hemicranial, and eye-focused. Source: Rogers Fund, 1910. Public Domain

Disorders 2020). CTH is a disabling and substantive condition, nonetheless, some nonpharmacological therapies are effective (Skelly et al. 2020).

Chronic migraine (CMH) may present with bilateral non-throbbing pain. CMH often requires prophylactic medication, especially in patients without a prior adequate trial of basic prophylactic medication, e.g. topiramate. Start with consistent application of basic headache and general pain principles. For both chronic tension headache and chronic migraine headache, careful examination of the head and neck for trigger points should be performed. Trigger points in the head, neck, or shoulders should prompt referral to a physical therapist enthusiastic about treating chronic headache. If a PT writes back that they don't know why you've referred the patient, seek out someone passionate about headaches. Many headaches are perpetuated by cervical and upper thoracic musculoskeletal abnormalities – this occurs by both central and peripheral pain mechanisms – controlling this is central to managing chronic headaches. Start prophylactic medication gradually.

Chronic daily headache (medication overuse headache) arises in patients taking daily analgesia. Over time, rebound or lowered pain-thresholds develop from chronic analgesia exposure; both acetaminophen and NSAIDs to some degree are implicated in these phenomena. The patient must be tapered from the agent that they are using too frequently, this may mean using alternative therapies, e.g. acupuncture, massage, meditation, physical therapy, TENS, prophylactic pharmacotherapy. The headaches will not likely resolve until the offending analgesic agent is eliminated from daily use.

Additional chronic headaches include trigeminal autonomic cephalalgias specifically cluster headaches, paroxysmal hemicranias, and SUNCT (short, unilateral, neuralgiform, corneal injection, and tearing) (Figure 42.2). Cluster headache and hemicranias are associated with behavioral agitation. The trigeminal autonomic headaches should be evaluated by imaging to exclude pituitary, hypothalamic, or mass lesions. These headaches manifest primarily in the V1 dermatomal area but C2, V2, and V3 may also be affected. Functional MRI indicates that there is activation of hypothalamic and brainstem nuclei in these disorders.

Cluster headache is much more prevalent in males where it manifests with very severe pain. Most often a stabbing or sharp pain retroorbitally, the sensation of pain is extreme and may provoke suicidal ideation. Behavioral agitation is frequent with pacing, groaning, or head-holding; parasympathetic or sympathetic perturbance is required for diagnosis. The headaches cluster, occurring daily for weeks followed by remissions of months to years. Triggers include alcohol, fumes, strenuous exercise, and sleep perturbance; smoking is common. A disturbance of the suprachiasmatic nucleus effecting circadian rhythms is postulated. Oxygen and SQ sumatriptan are potentially effective therapies.

Paroxysmal hemicrania is characterized by brief (12–15 minute) attacks of sharp unilateral headache multiple times daily. Autonomic features are present ipsilaterally. The episodic form affects males and females equally while the chronic form has a female predominance. The paroxysmal hemicranias are responsive to indomethacin.

Knowledge of common chronic headache types is very useful in primary care practice; and basic comprehensive management including pharmacological and non-pharmacological elements is necessary to limit the persistent disability and suffering associated with chronic headache.

References

Chung, F., Yegneswaran, B., Liao, P. et al. (2008). STOP questionnaire: a tool to screen patients for obstructive sleep apnea. Anesthesiology 108 (5): 812–821.

International Classification of Headache Disorders (2020). https://www.ichd-3.org/wp-content/uploads/2018/01/TheInternational-Classification-of-Headache-Disorders-3rd-Edition-2018.pdf (accessed 22 June 2020).

Klinger, R., Stuhlreyer, J., Schwartz, M. et al. (2018). Clinical use of placebo effects in patients with pain disorders. International Review of Neurobiology 139: 107–128.

Skelly, A.C., Chou, R., Dettori, J.R. et al. (2020). Noninvasive Nonpharmacological Treatment for Chronic Pain: A Systematic Review Update. Rockville, MD: Agency for Healthcare Research and Quality; 2020 Apr. Report No.: 20-EHC009. PMID: 32338846.

Visceral pain has features distinct from "somatic" pain. These include distinctive pain signaling molecules, and the perception of pain as diffuse, or referred. Referred pain is often perceived in a stereotypical location, e.g., cardiac ischemia causing left arm or jaw pain. It can have distinctive cramping or colicky temporal quality.

Anatomy and innervation

Visceral pain is signaled by some somatic pain neurotransmitters as well as special visceral mediators. Glutamate, CGRP, and protons, with receptors and channel proteins are also found in somatic nociceptors, e.g. TRPV1, ASIC3, and NaV1.8 (Yam et al. 2018). Opioid, endocannabinoid, and visceral inflammatory signals are also important. Sensory fibers from viscera transit para- or prevertebral ganglia before entering the spinal cord. The vagus nerve carries afferents from heart, lung, and GI structures via CN 10. GI structures from small intestine to midcolon have afferents via the celiac, superior, and inferior mesenteric ganglia, whereas distal colon and pelvic viscera project to lumbar and sacral cord via the pelvic ganglion. Many of these axons are thinly or unmyelinated, subserving diffuse pain sensation; they closely match those of the somatic pain system (CGRP is observed in lung and pancreas). (Mazzone and Undem 2016) In the gut, there is a semiautonomous enteric nervous system that regulates peristalsis (Meldgaard et al. 2019). This extensive network communicates with the central nervous system in a limited manner; contributing to limited gastrointestinal pain localization.

Referred pain is a common feature of visceral pain and of fundamental importance to clinical assessment (Figure 43.1). Pain referral is a poorly understood phenomenon, variously ascribed to visceral structures cosynapsing on second order neurons that also signal in response to somatic pain inputs, or to the minimal myelination and extensive presence of unmyelinated axons which might implicate interaxonal "crosstalk" (Figure 43.2). Some common referred pain patterns include cardiac pain radiating to left arm and jaw; esophageal pain radiating to the lower sternum, pancreatic pain to the center back; bladder to the low abdomen; and kidney and ureter to the flank (low lateral back, hip, and thigh area).

A final important feature of visceral pain is the **reflex arc** responses to noxious or painful sensory input. These include responses reflective of the function of the organ, e.g. capsaicin in the lung provokes bronchospasm. But also include reflex local muscle spasms that can lead to chronic pain syndromes. These were recognized by Barbara Travell, who observed trigger points in patients with cardiac and pulmonary disease and noted persistent pain. Identification and treatment of these trigger points did not alter the course of the underlying disease, but did alleviate a major source of suffering. Reflex arc functions can be of critical importance in thoracic visceral disease where reflex muscle contraction can lead to respiratory splinting with impaired oxygenation, atelectasis, and potentially pneumonia.

Common and relevant conditions

Acute visceral pain syndromes are among the most common conditions prompting people to seek medical attention, these include: myocardial infarction, cholecystitis, pancreatitis, appendicitis, renal stones, urinary tract infection, and diverticulitis. These are not detailed here but training for management of acute visceral pain is generally strong. Characterization of chest pain, central to general clinical training, is a good model for characterizing pain conditions – assessing *Q*uality, *R*egion, *S*everity, and *T*iming of pain, as well as the *U*sually-associated symptoms, alle*V*iating activities, and *W*orsening factors (Q-R-S-T and U-V-W of pain evaluation).

Notably, gender differences impact visceral pain beyond sex-specific organs (Dodds et al. 2016). Women can manifest cardiac ischemia atypically (Safdar and D'Onofrio 2016). Mortality from atypical chest pain is higher; clinicians should anticipate that women presenting with subacute chest *discomfort* require risk factor appraisal (age, family history of early MI) and assessment. Common chronic visceral pain syndromes are discussed here.

Esophagitis, common in adults, occurs in the young as well. Producing intermittent pain over the lower sternum; esophagitis arises from GERD, food allergies, and other causes (Esophagitis. Mayo Clinic 2020). Unchecked, lower esophageal inflammation can cause esophageal strictures or precancerous changes. While the upper esophagus demonstrates excellent sensory localization, in the lower esophagus localization is poor: esophagitis is associated with diffuse pain, referring to the chest wall at the lower sternum. Comprehensive management includes lifestyle changes, diet, avoidance of triggers, and medication.

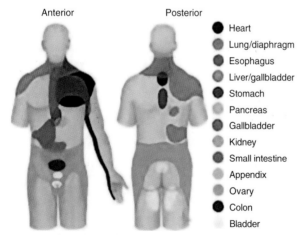

Anterior	Posterior

- Heart
- Lung/diaphragm
- Esophagus
- Liver/gallbladder
- Stomach
- Pancreas
- Gallbladder
- Kidney
- Small intestine
- Appendix
- Ovary
- Colon
- Bladder

Figure 43.1 Visceral pain often manifests with "referred pain," pain perceived in an area of the body that has a predictable pattern.

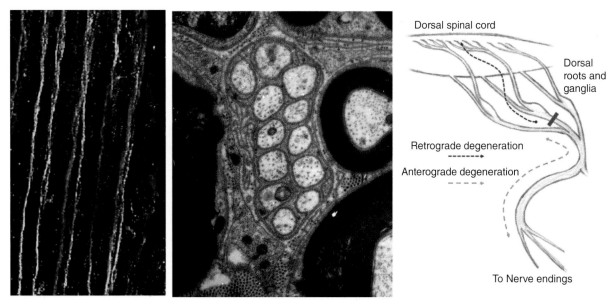

Figure 43.2 Peripheral and central structures may contribute to the phenomenon of referred pain. In this figure, juxtaposition of C-fiber (many pain-signaling) axons in peripheral nerve, and degeneration, injury, or highly active signaling of one may affect the other. Dorsal horn is also a site commonly noted a location of potential interaction between visceral and somatic structures.

Chronic pancreatitis, not uncommon, produces disabling, severe upper abdomen pain radiating to mid-back. Classically associated with alcohol consumption, not all persons with pancreatitis consume alcohol and stigmatization must be avoided (Kuhlmann et al. 2019). When chronic, the inflammation associated with pancreatitis can disrupt digestive enzyme production, unchecked the pancreas may deteriorate. Fatty stools, nutrient mal-absorption, and weight loss may ensue. Compassionate, compre-hensive management includes lifestyle changes, bowel rest, and specialist care (Singh and Drewes 2017).

Irritable bowel syndrome, highly prevalent, causes chronic periods of frequent abdominal pain and changes in bowel habits. Diarrhea, constipation, or alternating diarrhea and constipation (mixed pattern) occur. Long associated with chronic stress, data show bidirectional relationships between stress and lower GI bacteria (Moloney et al. 2015). GI viscera are strongly impacted by

local bacteria – microbial phenotyping shows microbes impact the inflammatory pain signaling in viscera (Vila et al. 2018). The gut serves as a barrier to materials ingested daily. In patients with IBS, the intestinal lining is semipermeable and inflammation ensues. IBS requires comprehensive management including changes to diet, stress reduction, use of probiotics, and in some, medication (Lee et al. 2019).

Interstitial cystitis (IC) produces symptoms of chronic bladder irritation: pain in the low abdomen and pelvis, and urinary urgency. Symptoms feel like a UTI but bacteria are not found and antibiotics are not recommended. IC is far more common in women, and exac-erbated by prolonged sitting, stress, and sexual activity. Persons with other chronic pain conditions have increased risk for IC. Comprehensive management includes urological evaluation, life-style management, and medications (Olesen et al. 2016). Tricyclic antidepressants may decrease urinary frequency and pain.

For references, please turn to page 108.

Although not unique to women, pelvic pain syndromes, with the exception of prostate pain, show a strong female predominance. Historically, pelvic pain has been stigmatized; it is important to respect cultural and personal perspectives towards the pelvic region while evincing a proactive, professional stance in assessing and addressing pelvic pain. Pelvic pain syndromes consist of nociceptive, inflammatory, and neuropathic pain syndromes that affect somatic, i.e. musculoskeletal, as well as visceral structures.

Anatomy and physiology

The pelvis consists of two ilium bones and the sacrum. The two ilia meet anteriorly at the symphysis pubis and connect to the sacrum posterolaterally (bilateral sacroiliac joints), painful dysfunction and arthritic change can occur (Figure 44.1). The pelvic bones anchor muscles involved in bounding the abdominal cavity and essential to ambulation, trigger points in these muscles, "external" to the pelvis may result in pain syndromes referring to the pelvis (Figure 44.2). The pelvic floor is comprised of multiple muscles the dysfunction of which contributes visceral dysfunction and pelvic pain. The pelvic structures and organs are innervated predominantly by nerves from sacral spinal levels but lumbar and coccygeal levels contribute.

Common and relevant conditions

Bladder pain is common and distressing. Simple UTI can produce transient profound pain with urination, and patients should be advised in the use of OTC analgesia for pain relief (Duke Health Blog, 2019). Chronic bladder pain is not uncommon, please see Chapter 43 for interstitial cystitis.

Prostatic pain (prostadynia) is not uncommon but diagnosed in only 1 in 10 000 older adult males; by contrast, prostatitis is much more common and is diagnosed in approximately 1% of males aged 65 and over – it is more common in younger men. **Prostatitis** produces frequent, painful urination; it can be caused by bacterial infection, pelvic trauma, catheter placement, pelvic dysfunction, or other infection including HIV (Mayo Clinic 2020). It may present with diffuse or referred pain in the low back, groin, external genitalia, or perineum. Following physical examination, urinalysis, and other tests, antibiotics may be used for bacterial infections, and alpha-adrenergic blockade or NSAIDs may ease symptoms. If chronic, comprehensive management includes avoidance of bladder-irritating foods (spicy foods, caffeine) limiting sitting, warm sitz baths, biofeedback, acupuncture, or dietary supplements.

Rectal pain can arise from multiple conditions, perhaps most feared being rectal adenocarcinoma. Benign causes of rectal pain are more common with hemorrhoids affecting a significant number of adults. Rectal pain necessitates evaluation. In most, avoidance of

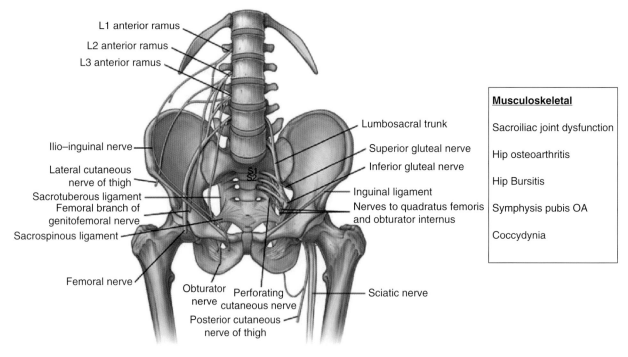

Musculoskeletal
Sacroiliac joint dysfunction
Hip osteoarthritis
Hip Bursitis
Symphysis pubis OA
Coccydynia

Figure 44.1 Skeletal anatomy of the pelvis with bones, ligaments, and lumbosacral nerve plexus. Source: Olayemi Kuponiyi MRCOG, et al. (2014). © John Wiley & Sons.

Pain Medicine at a Glance, First Edition. Beth B. Hogans.
© 2022 John Wiley & Sons Ltd. Published 2022 by John Wiley & Sons Ltd.

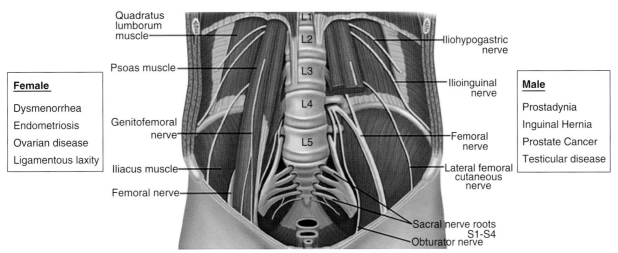

Quadratus lumborum muscle

Psoas muscle

Genitofemoral nerve

Iliacus muscle

Femoral nerve

L1
L2
L3
L4
L5

Iliohypogastric nerve

Ilioinguinal nerve

Femoral nerve

Lateral femoral cutaneous nerve

Sacral nerve roots S1–S4

Obturator nerve

Female

Dysmenorrhea

Endometriosis

Ovarian disease

Ligamentous laxity

Male

Prostadynia

Inguinal Hernia

Prostate Cancer

Testicular disease

Figure 44.2 Anatomy of posterior pelvic wall illustrating course of femoral, lateral femoral cutaneous, and obturator nerves, as well as sacral nerve roots and plexus. Source: Olayemi Kuponiyi MRCOG, et al. (2014). © John Wiley & Sons.

constipation is vitally important. Other useful measures can be the use of donut cushions and small cool packs for comfort.

Musculoskeletal pelvic pain is common. Perhaps the most common is sacroiliac dysfunction (Chapter 35). The anterior pelvic symphysis is located at the center of the anterior pelvic rim; it can become acutely painful in mid-to-late pregnancy (Chapter 53). Later in life, some experience chronic arthritic pain of the pelvic joints. Trigger points in the interior pelvic muscles can cause chronic pelvic pain; knowledge of these syndromes and access to specialty gyn-PT care impact syndrome resolution.

Primary dysmenorrhea is pain associated with menstruation; **secondary dysmenorrhea** is secondary to other conditions such as uterine fibroids, endometriosis, or adenomyosis. Primary dysmenorrhea typically responds to basic analgesia care or with hormonal modulation, i.e. oral contraceptives (Cleveland Clinic Foundation 2020). Basic analgesia for primary dysmenorrhea should begin, unless specific reasons contravene, with ibuprofen. A fast-acting formulation of ibuprofen is ibuprofen sodium, demonstrated in meta-analysis to provide faster, more effective, and more durable analgesia for dysmenorrhea and other common pain-associated conditions. It is worthwhile to titrate therapy upwards rather than immediately instituting an 800 mg dose. Comprehensive management includes physical activity in the inter-catamenial period, ensuring sufficient rest, mitigating stress, and encouraging hydration; acupuncture, yoga, and mindfulness may help.

Endometriosis and **pelvic congestion syndrome** may cause chronic pelvic pain. Endometriosis, a chronic inflammatory process, produces fluctuating pain with pain commencing before the menstrual cycle and persisting afterwards. Pelvic congestion syndrome is a vascular phenomenon with high prevalence, approaching 10% in middle-aged women (Osman et al. 2013). It is associated with chronic pain including deep, aching pelvic pain referring to the low back, without reference to the menstrual cycle but worsened with prolonged standing, coitus, pregnancy, or fatigue.

Vaginismus is a syndrome of painful muscle spasm in the pelvic floor affecting the vagina, worsened with actual or attempted pen-

etration either during sexual activity or even tampon use. This is a complex condition that requires specialist care, and coordinated comprehensive care is typical.

Vulvodynia is a syndrome of pain of the external female urogenitalia; it is provoked by contact, touching, or pressure. The mechanisms of vulvodynia are principally thought to be neuropathic. Treatment should be comprehensive and follow an appropriate evaluation. Pharmacological options may include tricyclic antidepressants, topical agents, and others.

Pelvic muscle trigger points are an important source of chronic pain for women. The treatments for pelvic muscle trigger points can require accessing the interior of the pelvis through the vagina, and it is important to seek out expert treatment and assure the patient's safety during this process. Given that major muscles controlling the legs originate on the back wall of the pelvis, i.e. iliopsoas, and the multiplicity of pelvic muscles and demands placed on them, the development of trigger points is not entirely surprising. With some patients, it is possible for them to learn approaches to self-treatment; nonetheless, this may not be effective in all situations.

References

Cleveland Clinic Foundation (2020). Dysmenorrhea. https://my.clevelandclinic.org/health/diseases/4148-dysmenorrhea#:~:text=Secondary%20dysmenorrhea%20is%20pain%20that,longer%20than%20common%20menstrual%20cramps (accessed 11 August 2020).

Duke Health Blog (2019). Tracking down relief for a urinary tract infection. https://www.dukehealth.org/blog/tracking-down-relief-urinary-tract-infection (accessed 11 August 2020).

Mayo Clinic (2020). Prostatitis. https://www.mayoclinic.org/diseases-conditions/prostatitis/diagnosis-treatment/drc-20355771 (accessed 11 August 2020).

Osman, M.W., Nikolopoulos, I., Jayaprakasan, K., and Raine-Fenning, N. (2013). Pelvic congestion syndrome. *The Obstetrician & Gynaecologist* 15: 151–157.

45 Exceptional causes of severe, chronic pain: CRPS, fibromyalgia, erythromelalgia, and small fiber peripheral neuropathy

Several conditions are well-known as severe chronic pain conditions; among these are chronic regional pain syndrome (CRPS), fibromyalgia, and erythromelalgia. The actual incidence of CRPS and erythromelalgia is extremely low, but because patients with these conditions comprise part of academic pain practice, these conditions are emphasized in medical school teaching programs. Conditions such as low back pain, headache, knee pain, and others are vastly more common in primary care practice (Murphy et al. 2017) and yet receive very little attention in traditional education (Mezei et al. 2011). One relatively common cause of severe chronic pain is small fiber neuropathy, most often arising from diabetes or prediabetes, but potentially due to other causes. Finally, congenital insensitivity to pain is also discussed here.

CRPS is a chronic, severely painful condition known since the U.S. Civil War (Mitchell, 1872). The ballistic injuries that occurred were associated with advances in medicine that resulted in wounded soldiers surviving, but with injuries that sometimes developed into chronic pain. At the present time, CRPS is classified into type I and type II where type II is associated with demonstrable injury to nerve and type I is not associated with clear nerve injury. A series of changes are observable with CRPS – an early phase with edema, erythema, and increased temperature of the involved limb, Figure 45.1a. This is followed over several months, by a late (atrophic) phase associated with pallor, cooling, and bone demineralization. In both phases, patients report excruciating levels of pain including allodynia, i.e. exquisite pain in response to light touch or cold air. Patients may wear special coverings over the affected limb. This should be discouraged as it may worsen the syndrome. In some patients, the pain is sympathetically mediated, demonstrable through relief with sympathetic blockade but this is not currently utilized in routine clinical practice. In preclinical studies, pentoxyphylline has been utilized to block inflammatory mediators, such as TNF-alpha (Wei et al. 2009). The injury that precipitates CRPS is a peripheral injury, but pathological changes occur in both peripheral and central nervous systems. At this point in time, there is no definitive treatment that can prevent or reverse these changes, but researchers are working toward this goal. One possibility is to quickly block nerves to an injury site, which may reduce the development of CRPS. Former names for CRPS include causalgia and reflex sympathetic dystrophy.

Fibromyalgia is a disorder of pain in many parts of the body simultaneously. For many years, the diagnosis was based on tenderness provoked by palpation at specified locations on the body (Petzke et al. 2003). In 2010, new diagnostic criteria were promulgated: widespread pain (multiple sites) with generalized fatigue, waking unrefreshed, and cognitive symptoms, as well as other symptoms (Wolfe et al. 2010). There is some controversy about the mechanisms causing fibromyalgia (Gracely et al. 2002). It is important to ensure the patient does not have other conditions that explain the symptoms: poly-arthritis; sleep apnea, highly prevalent in men (24%) and women (9%); hypothyroidism; cervical myelopathy; lupus; Ehlers–Danlos syndrome; and rheumatoid arthritis may mimic fibromyalgia (Garvey et al. 2015). Reliance on opioids is inappropriate in these patients. Milnacipran, an antidepressant in Europe, is potentially effective (Mease et al. 2009). Comprehensive management is essential, especially moderate daily exercise (Skelly et al. 2020).

Fabry's disease is a rare X-linked glycogen storage disorder that results in a syndrome of lancinating pains. There are hundreds of peripheral nerve conditions, many with pain. A valuable resource for these is the neuromuscular disease website located at Washington University at Saint Louis. Thousands of diseases of the nervous system from rare to common are documented: http://neuromuscular.wustl.edu.

Erythromelalgia is a dramatic condition for which specific mechanisms have been identified (Dib-Hajj et al. 2005). A mutation in one of the voltage-dependent sodium channel genes can produce this syndrome, characterized by episodic severe pain accompanied by intense reddening of the extremities, (Kim et al. 2013) Figure 45.1b and c.

The inability to sense pain, i.e. **congenital insensitivity to pain** is exceedingly rare. There are multiple gene defects producing this phenotype, the first person definitively identified was a "double heterozygote" who received distinctly mutated genes for SCN9A from each parent – this person did not experience pain in response

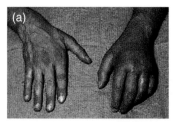 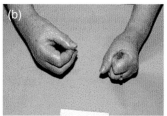 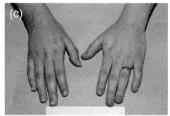 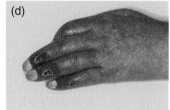

Figure 45.1 (a) Early phase CRPS: the left hand is edematous, discolored and shows atrophic skin changes; (b) erythromelalgia: transient episodes of severe pain and intense reddening of the feet, (c) baseline pale coloration of the same patient.

Pain Medicine at a Glance, First Edition. Beth B. Hogans.
© 2022 John Wiley & Sons Ltd. Published 2022 by John Wiley & Sons Ltd.

to trauma, and ultimately died accidentally (Cox et al. 2006). It is notable that one mutation of the SCN9 gene produces erythromelalgia (gain-of-function syndrome), while a complimentary mutation produces a loss-of-function (congenital insensitivity to pain).

Much more common by far but often unrecognized is **small fiber peripheral neuropathy (SFN)**. This condition involves selective degeneration of C-fibers, many of which are pain-sensing. Patients often experience distressing burning pain but do not have any other signs easily identified on standard examination (Marchettini et al. 2006). Muscle strength, reflexes, light touch, vibration testing, and position sense testing and all other parts of the neurological examination are usually normal. It can be very frustrating for these patients to experience disabling pain, and be told that "nothing seems to be wrong." One key exam abnormality is the elicitation of sharp hyperalgesia – observable through special testing: repeated tapping on distal foot with a sharp probe (a broken wood applicator, not a safety pin) at about 3x/second is normally minimally bothersome, Figure 45.2, but patients with SFN experience rapidly amplifying intense pain. About half of people with diabetes will develop peripheral neuropathy, many selectively affecting small fibers; in about half of these, the neuropathy is painful, others will experience numbness, non-painful pressure, or phantom sensations. Testing is described in Figure 45.3 and includes bloodwork and skin biopsy for nerve fiber (PGP9.5 antigen) testing, and in some cases sural nerve biopsy (Murinson 2006), Figure 45.4. Treatment usually includes strict diabetes control, if relevant, treatment of other causative conditions, potential repletion of vitamin B_{12}, footcare and medications such as gabapentinoids.

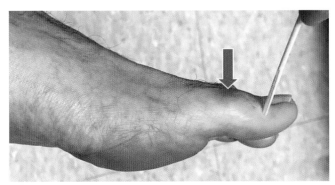

Figure 45.2 Tapping distal phalanx of great toe with a sharp stick to test sharp sensation; tapping quickly (3 Hz) to elicit hyperalgesia. Blue arrow indicates demarcation between distal and proximal toe.

Potential cause	Testing
Diabetes or impaired glucose tolerance	2 hour glucose tolerance test
Lyme disease	Lyme test
Lupus	ANA
Rheumatoid arthritis	Rheumatoid factor
Sarcoidosis	ACE
Renal or hepatic impairment	Chemistries: Creatinine, AST/ALT

Figure 45.3 Potential causes and preliminary testing for small fiber neuropathy. Leprosy more common than diabetes or Lyme disease in some regions.

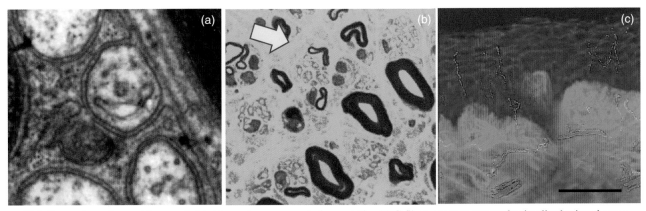

Figure 45.4 Comparison of nerve biopsy and skin biopsy for assessment of neuropathy. (a) C-fibers are most accurately visualized using electron microscopy, not feasibly employed for routine clinical assessment, and (b) sometimes visualizable using light microscopy of nerve biopsy, yellow arrow, but not reliably for clinical testing; by contrast, immunochemical staining of 3 mm skin punch biopsy samples (c) is now well-validated to quantitatively evaluate unmyelinated nerve fibers in skin, samples can be taken at multiple locations, e.g. distal ankle and proximal hip, providing evidence of length-dependent (dying back) neuropathy. Nerve biopsy is still used to evaluate some causes of neuropathy including vasculitis, amyloid, leprosy, or sarcoidosis. Bars are 1 μm (a), 10 μm (b), 100 μm (c).

For references, see page 108.

Caring for those with substance abuse disorders and pain can be highly rewarding; in the ideal, you work closely with the patient to build trust, focus on recovery, and make healthy choices that will, with time and effort, bring pain under control. The path of the provider and the patient can nonetheless be eventful: the management of pain in patients with comorbid pain conditions and substance use disorders is complex for multiple reasons (Figure 46.1). One central complication is the alteration of pain processing in those with opioid use disorder and the impact of substance use generally on mental health. Severe and chronic pain deeply challenge mental well-being, even the healthiest person from a mental and emotional standpoint will be sorely tested when experiencing high impact, chronic pain. For the patient with substance use disorder and pain simultaneously, a coordinated multiprofessional support team working together utilizing interprofessional skills of teamwork, communication, roles and responsibilities, and values is necessary.

Patients with substance use disorder respond best to comprehensive management, not dissimilar from comprehensive management for chronic pain conditions. The challenge is finding therapies that compliment these dual comorbidities – without overwhelming.

Provider safety is not negotiable at any time in healthcare. Your life cannot be threatened or endangered as you render care to patients, period. Before agreeing to take care of patients with pain, evaluate the safety context of your practice setting. Before agreeing to prescribe opioids or take care of patients with substance use disorders and chronic pain, require a professional discussion of safety measures – these can include having a silent alarm, having a panic button, having a security guard available and on premises, having a clinic room with two entrances, having a rear entrance to the clinic for providers, having a chaperone for some or all clinic visits, having training for all staff on recognizing the signs of patient stress and de-escalation of fraught interactions. Tapering opioids or managing pain in the context of SUD is highly stressful

for patients, there will be times when patients become annoyed, aggravated, angry, hostile, threatening, violent, homicidal, or suicidal. If you are prepared and practiced in your responses, it is less likely that hazardous conduct will occur. Make sure to maintain strong and positive channels of communication with all staff, have a clear chain of responsibility, monitor for staff-splitting behaviors, e.g., "I don't like your on-call partner, he lied to me about calling in a prescription when my pills fell in the toilet," and take time to appreciate others and celebrate therapeutic successes.

Patients with substance abuse disorders are preferably in recovery and supported by a regular, stable mental health provider in order to engage effectively in comprehensive pain management. You must have clear policies about whether opioids will be prescribed. Do not be surprised that patients who expect opioids become angry when learning that opioids will not be prescribed (Figure 46.2). Do not be disappointed when a patient who has just engaged in a 20 minute conversation about yoga and meditation ends the visit with a request for oxycodone. Your affect cannot be determined by theirs – even when you meet them part way in order to empathize and foster rapport. Clear interpersonal boundaries and prior expectations (for yourself) and effectively documented "informed consent" for the patient to receive pain treatments are essential (Figure 46.3).

With all the evidence supporting the need for patients with SUD or in recovery to realize the maximum possible benefit from non-pharmacological therapies, surprisingly little is known about the extent to which chronic opioid exposure impacts the efficacy of nonpharmacological therapies (Substance Abuse and Mental Health Services Administration (SAMHSA) 2016). Acupuncture, moderate daily exercise, and yoga may all be modulated by endogenous opioids. Consider the impact of chronic corticosteroid

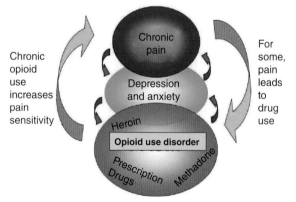

Figure 46.1 There is a complex interplay between pain, substance use disorders, and mental health, these interactions are not well understood but have major implications for clinical care and decision-making, increasing the complexity of encounters and raising potential for harm.

Gender
Family history of substance abuse
Alcohol
Illegal drugs
Prescription drugs
Personal history of substance abuse
Alcohol
Illegal drugs
Prescription drugs
Age: 16—45 years
History of preadolescent sexual abuse
Psychological disease
ADD, OCD, bipolar, schizophrenia
Depression

Figure 46.2 Opioid risk tool elements.

Pain Medicine at a Glance, First Edition. Beth B. Hogans.
© 2022 John Wiley & Sons Ltd. Published 2022 by John Wiley & Sons Ltd.

Activity	Analgesia
Mobility	Pain intensity on average
Ability to work, school	Pain intensity at worst
Sleep	How often does pain reach
Relationships: family. friends	maximum intensity
Enjoyment of life	Change in quality or location

Adverse effects	Abuse/aberrant behavior
Constipation	Urine drug-tox failure/refusal
Nausea, Vomiting	Lost or stolen prescription
Cognitive decline, clouding	Request for name brand
Loss of libido	Behavior or appearance
Weight loss or gain	Dose escalation w/o consultation
Sleep disruption, fatigue	Refusal of nonpharm. treatment

Figure 46.3 The four A's of balanced analgesia: It is important to assess and balance the anticipated benefits: increased activity and Analgesia with the potential harms of treatment: Adverse effects and Abuse/aberrant behavior.

Resting pulse rate
GI upset
Sweating
Tremor
Restlessness
Yawning
Pupil dilation
Anxiety-Irritability
Bone/joint aches
Runny nose/tearing
Gooseflesh skin

Figure 46.4 Elements of COWS assessment for opioid withdrawal (Clinical Opioid Withdrawal Scale File 2009).

administration on endogenous adrenal-axis function – we know that chronic opioid exposure causes a downregulation of opioid receptors, effectively making it more difficult for each molecule of opioid-medication to find and bind to an available receptor.

Chronic opioid exposure causes lasting changes in the pain processing system. Persons with chronic opioid exposure have been shown to have lower pain thresholds, lower pain tolerance, and higher pain ratings. This is critically important to know and accept – the patient with opioid use disorder or licit chronic opioid exposure who appears to be exaggerating their pain, whether to venipuncture or other trauma from large to small, may actually be having a lived experience of markedly amplified pain (Opioid withdrawal Scales 2009) (Figure 46.4). For this reason, and all the special circumstances that pertain to patients with SUD, it is vitally important to utilizing comprehensive pain treatment approaches and be part of an interprofessional team when managing pain in those with SUD (Webster and Webster 2005).

Few conditions are as relentless as withdrawal and recovery from substance use. Even when the withdrawal is not fatal, the perceptions and experiences of the person going through the process are profound and often overwhelming. One treatment that may be especially helpful to the person overcoming a pain problem while living in recovery from SUD is the presence of a support animal or service animal. For many people, support animals provide moment-to-moment real contact with another living being. Living with a creature that perceives mood, and responds appropriately while empathizing and protecting can be a life-changing experience.

Despite all the challenges of providing pain care for those with or in recover from SUD, there is tremendous alignment of goals: utilizing all available resources to design and actively engage in healthy lifestyles and stress management are central to success (SAMHSA 2020).

References

Clinical Opioid Withdrawal Scale file:///C:/Users/Owner/Downloads/annex10-fm3.pdf Copyright © 2009, World Health Organization. Geneva All rights reserved. Publications of the World Health Organization can be obtained from WHO Press, World Health Organization, 20 Avenue Appia, 1211 Geneva 27, Switzerland (tel.: +41 22 791 3264; fax: +41 22 791 4857; e-mail: tni.ohw@sredrokoob). Requests for permission to reproduce or translate WHO publications – whether for sale or for noncommercial distribution – should be addressed to WHO Press, at the above address (fax: +41 22 791 4806; e-mail: tni.ohw@snoissimrep).

Opioid withdrawal Scales (2009) https://www.ncbi.nlm.nih.gov/books/NBK143183/ (accessed 14 August 2020).

Substance Abuse and Mental Health Services Administration (SAMHSA) (2016). Decisions in Recovery: Medications for Opioid Use Disorder. [Electronic Decision Support Tool] (HHS Pub No. SMA-16-4993), 2016. http://www.samhsa.gov/brss-tacs/shared-decision-making (accessed 14 August 2020).

Substance Abuse and Mental Health Services Administration (SAMHSA) (2020). The Opioid Crisis and the Black/African American Population: An Urgent Issue. Publication No. PEP20-05-02-001. Office of Behavioral Health Equity. Substance Abuse and Mental Health Services Administration.

Webster, L.R. and Webster, R. (2005). Predicting aberrant behaviors in Opioid-treated patients: preliminary validation of the Opioid risk too. Pain Medicine 6 (6): 432. https://www.drugabuse.gov/sites/default/files/opioidrisktool.pdf.

Palliative care addresses pain at the end of life as well as other symptomatic management and whole-person care (Providence Healthcare 2020) (Figure 47.1). Patients with life-limiting illness worry deeply about experiencing and dying with uncontrolled pain. Comprehensive pain management requires awareness that patients also experience high rates of other symptoms. These additional symptoms vary by individual and by stage-in-dying (Figure 47.2). For example, in patients with distressing dyspnea not addressable by other measures, opioids for pain may also relieve air hunger; by contrast, problematic constipation would be worsened by opioids.

Patients receiving end-of-life care often have prominent spiritual, emotional, and interpersonal needs and comprehensive pain management should be implemented utilizing an **interprofessional**

Pain
Dyspnea
Fatigue
Anorexia
Cachexia
Constipation
Diarrhea
Nausea/vomiting
Poorly healing wounds
Pressure sores
Anxiety
Depression
PTSD
Alterations of consciousness
Confusion
Delirium
Agitation

Figure 47.1 Many symptoms are associated with end-of-life; pain is the most feared.

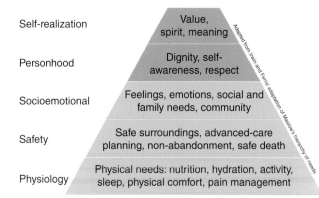

Figure 47.3 Patients have many needs, as exemplified by the layers shown here, an adaptation of Maslow's hierarchy of needs. The idea communicated by the "pyramid" is that patient's cannot explore the "higher levels" of needs unless the foundational needs for physiology and safety are met adequately.

team-based approach (Figure 47.3). The palliative care team includes physicians, nurses, pharmacists, physical therapist, occupational therapists, psychologists, social workers, clergy, and others.

One of the most powerful antidotes to pain is having a sense of **meaning in life**. Even though someone is nearing the end of their life, that time may be highly meaningful with interactions, essential tasks, meaningful conversations, and connection – others may need to have their privacy – in each case, dying is a highly personal experience (National ELNEC Project Team 2017). Pain should be controlled in a balanced manner so that alertness is preserved as long as the patient desires and such is possible.

An important aspect of caring for people with end-of-life pain has to do with the **barriers to care** and ensuring quality of care.

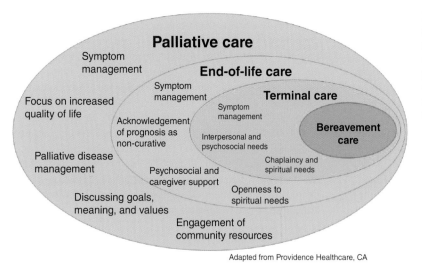

Adapted from Providence Healthcare, CA

Figure 47.2 Palliative care occurs as a spectrum from focusing of symptom-management, ideally prior to terminal diagnosis. Focus on symptom management is consistent but techniques vary according to patient preferences, stage, and context. Clinical, psychosocial, and spiritual needs persist at all phases, and comprehensive management (Chapter 16), modified according to patient tolerance and values is appropriate.

Pain Medicine at a Glance, First Edition. Beth B. Hogans.
© 2022 John Wiley & Sons Ltd. Published 2022 by John Wiley & Sons Ltd.

A recent study examined the perceptions of families and loved ones of patients receiving palliative care in a low resource environment. Those surveyed identified major deficiencies in accessing care as well as distress from healthcare provider attitudes and communication. One caregiver described the experience of taking her mother to hospice: ". . .she had to lie down in the back (of the car),. . .she was heavy set and even when we reach here, I had to take her out. The nurses couldn't and they were like, 'Yuh didn't bring a man with you?' (B88)" (Cox-Seignoret and Maharaj 2020). It is essentially important to engage social work and seek resources, including the support of significant others, friends, family, and volunteer organizations. Severe, unmitigated pain completely ruins every moment of the patient's remaining days and destroys the loved ones' hopes for a "peaceful death": "Caregivers described health professionals who seemed reluctant to prescribe opioids, delayed administration until late and utilized ineffective dosages. . .. '. . .we did not know that the pain was going to be so bad that there was nothing in this world that we could try that will help it. . . (N233)'" (Cox-Seignoret and Maharaj 2020).

Some states have legalized self-administration of prescribed medications causing death. This raises several ethical issues, but the presence of depression and other psychosocial factors can distort decision-making around end-of-life (Irwin and Ferris 2008). Providers must have a strong sense of how they apply ethics in caring for others as well as local legal constraints, but readily seek guidance when questions arise (see Chapter 10 for pain-related healthcare ethics) (Brummett (2020). A related issue is the phenomenon known as **double effect**: when a treatment for symptom-control produces changes in bodily functions that potentially diminish viability. Perspectives on double effect vary and practitioners should seek local ethical guidance. It is critically important to know and document patient's preferences in terms of pain management – and neither neglect the patient in pain nor terminate life early due to personal perspectives on what constitutes a life worth continuing (Cook and Rocker 2014). Patients are remarkably diverse – our duty is to strive to correctly manifest their interests, to the extent feasible and appropriate in delivering care (Agarwal and Murinson 2012).

Opioid rotation

Opioid rotation is a change in prescribed opioid medication intended to improve pain control and mitigate side effects. A recent systematic review examining opioid rotation in the context of cancer pain management found evidence to support the use of rotations to gain control over pain; most patients felt that the rotation was positive (Schuster et al. 2018). In the systematic review, it was noted that additional titration was necessary to attain pain control following rotation. With rotation, the dose of the second opioid is usually reduced below that calculated from equianalgesic tables. This is done for safety on the principle that cross-tolerance is less than 100%. There are some differences in opinion regarding whether and how much to reduce the dose of the second opioid – there is evidence that the dose will need to be titrated over the first 14 days following the change, and generally, except for methadone,

the titration is upwards. Although methadone may produce less constipation than other opioids, methadone as a pain agent is high risk. The analgesic effects of methadone have a shorter half-life than the respiratory suppression effects. For this reason, when methadone is titrated for pain treatment, exceptional care is needed – methadone should not be used for pain outside the context of an experienced pain service or provider with relevant advanced training. Fentanyl has also been used as an opioid that may not produce severe constipation; however, it may not be initiated in opioid-naïve patients, and it must be prescribed with care by an experienced, trained provider. Due to the variation in regional practices, specific rotation dosages should follow the established recommendations for each locality and facility.

The dissemination of knowledge and expertise pertaining to palliative care has been advanced by a train-the-trainer curriculum in palliative care called the End-of-Life Nursing education curriculum (**ELNEC**). ELNEC materials have undergone extensive development and are authoritatively referenced. Specialized ELNEC content addresses the needs of various populations including: pediatric patients, geriatric patients, and veterans.

References

Agarwal, A.K. and Murinson, B.B. (2012). New dimensions in patient-physician interaction: values, autonomy, and medical information in the patient-centered clinical encounter. Rambam Maimonides Medical Journal 3 (3): e0017. https://doi.org/10.5041/RMMJ.10085.

Brummett, A.L. (2020). Should positive claims of conscience receive the same protection as negative claims of conscience? Clarifying the asymmetry debate. The Journal of Clinical Ethics 31 (2): 136–142.

Cook, D. and Rocker, G. (2014). Dying with dignity in the intensive care unit. The New England Journal of Medicine 370: 2506–2514.

Cox-Seignoret, K. and Maharaj, R.G. (2020). Unmet needs of patients with cancer in their last year of life as described by caregivers in a developing world setting: a qualitative study. BMC Palliative Care 19 (1): 13. Published 24 January 2020. doi:https://doi.org/10.1186/s12904-020-0516-4.

Irwin, S.A. and Ferris, F.D. (2008). The opportunity for psychiatry in palliative care. Canadian Journal of Psychiatry 53 (11): 713–724.

National ELNEC Project Team (2017). Symptom Management, Module 3 in Faculty Guide for ELNEC-For Veterans END-OF-LIFE NURSING EDUCATION CONSORTIUM Palliative Care For Veterans. https://www.wehonorveterans.org/wp-content/uploads/2020/02/Mod3_FacultyGuide.pdf (accessed 29 June 2020).

Providence Healthcare (2020). What is Palliative Care?. http://hpc.providencehealthcare.org/about/what-palliative-care (accessed 16 August 2020).

Schuster, M., Bayer, O., Heid, F., and Laufenberg-Feldmann, R. (2018). Opioid Rotation in Cancer Pain Treatment. Deutsches Ärzteblatt International 115 (9): 135–142. https://doi.org/10.3238/arztebl.2018.0135. PMID: 29563006; PMCID: PMC5876542.

48 Opioids for chronic pain: preventing iatrogenic opioid use disorders

For many decades, controls on prescribing, distribution, and dispensing were so strict that patients with terminal cancer in the U.S. endured unbearable pain at the end of life. Then opioids became popular as therapy for acute and chronic noncancer pain (Figure 20.2). Increased prescribing contributed to widespread opioid dependence and many deaths ensued. In 2016, the CDC released evidence-based guidelines to prevent iatrogenic OUD (Dowell et al. 2016).

Because opioids are intensely reinforcing for many people, risks of dependence and misuse are serious (Figure 48.1). Guidance for safe opioid prescribing is based in best clinical practices, some suggested practice standards are highlighted here.

First: only prescribe opioids to patients you have examined and for whom you've established a reasoned differential diagnosis with a leading diagnosis appropriate to opioids. The evaluation should include weighing the risks and hazards of comorbidities. Many conditions and situations make opioids more harmful: chronic respiratory disease, alcohol abuse, concurrent benzodiazepines, CNS depressants, chronic constipation, substance use disorders, personality disorders (borderline personality), suicidality or depression, or someone in the home with active substance use (diversion risk). Taken as a whole, the patient must be appropriate for opioid therapy (Table 48.1).

Second: never prescribe opioids without also implementing a comprehensive pain management plan. If the patient refuses to participate in comprehensive care, e.g., physical therapy, group exercise, clinical psychology, meditation, etc., do not prescribe opioids. You set the standards and expectations and should do so clearly and before prescribing. If a patient refuses comprehensive management, incorporate this into your professional decision regarding whether opioids are appropriate and safe for the patient. You have many tools

Table 48.1 Potential harms and benefits of opioids.

Factors and health conditions that increase the potential harms of opioids
Chronic respiratory disease
Alcohol abuse
Concurrent benzodiazepines
Concurrent CNS depressants
Chronic constipation
Substance use disorders
Personality disorders (borderline personality)
Suicidality or depression

Potential benefits of opioids
Temporary relief of severe pain not amenable to other treatments

in your pain toolbox. Patients cannot demand "opioid-only" therapy – it is not safe, it is not correct. Train your support staff to explain before scheduling the first appointment that a comprehensive approach is used – including both medication and non-medication therapies. You can inform the patient at the first visit that you do not prescribe opioids in the absence of an established relationship, or until "all other" therapies have been tried. Finally, you may consider whether you won't prescribe opioids at all; however, there are patients with chronic pain-associated conditions who benefit from modest doses. Before you make a final decision about including opioids in your practice, check your organizational, local, and national professional standards.

Third: avoid opioid escalation. If you are considering an increase in opioid dose for your patient, check to make sure that you are within guidelines. Then optimize all other therapies – try a new form of non-pharmacological therapy, e.g. acupuncture, massage, hypnosis, cognitive behavioral therapy, acceptance commitment therapy, occupational therapy – try several new therapies, and retry previous therapies that seemed somewhat effective (perhaps with a new therapist). You can return to previously attempted nonopioid medications, barring allergy. Patients can resist nonopioid options. If they ask: "why do you think this medicine will work when it didn't help before?" A good answer is: "You are in a different place now – your pain-condition has changed over time, and as you've engaged some of the other therapies that we've been incorporating into your pain self-management plan, your pain system has changed – you might be more responsive to the medication now. We know that this medication works on the body's pain system and

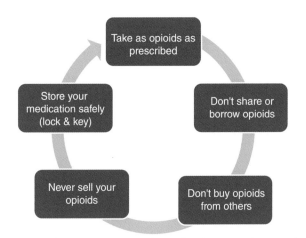

Figure 48.1 Can your patient or their caregiver be expected to meet the following behavioral requirements? What is the safety plan?

Pain Medicine at a Glance, First Edition. Beth B. Hogans.
© 2022 John Wiley & Sons Ltd. Published 2022 by John Wiley & Sons Ltd.

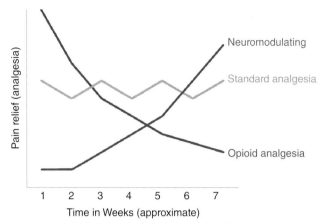

Figure 48.2 Opioids have a decline in analgesic efficacy over time that is a predictable and expected component of their action. By contrast, standard OTC analgesics, like ibuprofen, demonstrate consistent analgesia (given stable pain), and neuromodulating agents, especially pain-active antidepressant, increase in effect over time. The figure illustrates this graphically.

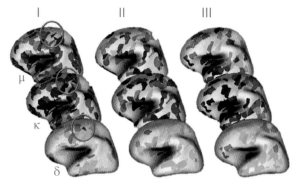

Figure 48.3 Opioids have multiple receptors that manifest different properties. People are quite diverse in terms of the expression of these receptor types. The brains below represent the density of immunochemical identification of three main opioid receptor types, Mu, Kappa, and Delta (μ, κ, and δ) in the brains of three different individuals, labeled here: I, II, and III. The receptors vary from person to person in absolute and relative amounts. Adapted from the Allen Brain Atlas.

it is reasonable to think that it could help. We know that it is safer than increasing the opioid." Opioids have an inherent property of tolerance, once you make the decision to increase the dose, you will likely be chasing pain relief that is fleeting, but dependence will be lasting (Figure 48.2).

Fourth: Do not prescribe or promise such until you have personally checked the prescription database monitoring program (PDMP) data (CDC 2016). PDMP data have appropriately levelled the playing field for providers prescribing controlled substances. Prior to PDMP implementation, providers were burdened – who could call all the pharmacies in a major metropolitan area to check for other prescribers? – those patients determined to evade detection could do so. With the PDMP, providers have access to appropriate clinical details – increasing safety for all patients.

Guidance for opioid prescribing was described several years ago as "Universal precautions for Opioids"; except for shifts away from "treatment contracts" towards "informed consent for treatment," these precautions remain generally useful (Gourlay et al. 2005).

The risks of opioids are well established: Some patients will develop disordered opioid use when drugs are first encountered in a licit medical context. We have limited capacity to predict which patients are at most risk but some risk assessment techniques are available. One of these is the **Opioid Risk Tool** (Chapter 46). The patient has completed the questions, the provider scores them, and this estimates risk. The higher the score, the higher the risk of misuse or abuse.

With all the considerations against utilizing opioids, there are some patients who appear to benefit from stable daily doses, it is not known what percentage of the population responds well to opioid therapy (Figure 48.3). Even still, there is limited information regarding extended long-term benefits of opioid therapy – most clinical studies have only examined pain relief over a time-course of weeks. Finally, a few carefully selected patients can effectively use opioids on a nonescalating as needed basis for the relief of pain flares. In this case, the provider has addressed all of the above concerns. In general, a prescription providing for three doses of opioid per week may be a useful opioid rescue strategy that avoids excessive induction of tolerance. Although seemingly prudent, clinical trials are still needed to validate this approach.

References

CDC (2016). Prescription Drug Monitoring Programs (PDMPs): What States Need to Know. https://www.cdc.gov/drugoverdose/pdmp/states.html (accessed 13 August 2020).

Dowell, D., Haegerich, T.M., and Chou, R.C.D.C. (2016). Guideline for prescribing opioids for chronic pain — United States, 2016. MMWR - Recommendations and Reports 65 (RR-1): 1–49. https://doi.org/10.15585/mmwr.rr6501e1.

Gourlay, D.L., Heit, H.A., and Almahrezi, A. (2005). Universal precautions in pain medicine: a rational approach to the treatment of chronic pain. Pain Medicine 6 (2): 107–112.

49 Tapering opioids in patients with pain

Tapering opioids in patients with pain is a fundamental skill in the management of pain. Opioid withdrawal is associated with multiple unpleasant symptoms as well as a marked increase in lived pain experience – in those with established pain-associated conditions, rapid opioid tapering may be unendurably awful, and suicides have been reported (Table 49.1).

In patients with chronic pain who have been treated with opioids for relatively long periods of time, the preferred approach to opioid tapering is to do a very slow taper. In fact, the most tolerable approach may feel excruciatingly slow to the provider who is not familiar with the difficulties associated with opioid withdrawal. Opioid withdrawal has many unpleasant symptoms, (Table 49.1), but the most problematic for those with chronic pain is the profound exacerbation of the lived pain experience that occurs for most patients. Some will use illicit or unregulated opioids to relieve pain and providers should be vigilant for signs of overdose (Table 49.2).

There are three main scenarios in opioid tapering: (i) Both patient and provider agree that opioids are not beneficial and that taper is appropriate, (ii) Provider determines that side effects are problematic and that a taper is indicated and needs to be

undertaken at a pace that may be uncomfortable for the patient but that safety concerns predominate, and (iii) A major safety event has occurred, e.g., overdose, threatening words or behaviors, diversion, and ultra-rapid taper is required (Table 49.2). Each of these scenarios will be discussed (Table 49.3).

In the first scenario, the patient and provider agree that an opioid taper is appropriate for optimal care. This point may be reached through patient counseling – as the patient comes to understand the limitations of opioids for long-term pain management and the actual harms associated with opioids, and, as the patient begins to appreciate that nonpharmacological therapies and nonopioid medications are genuinely effective in managing pain – they reach the point that opioids are not preferred as a therapy (Els et al. 2017). This may take time or can occur for reasons that lie outside the patient–provider interaction, e.g. death of a family member due to opioid overdose. Barring side effects or acute risks due to opioids, the patient and provider can prepare and plan for opioid tapering together. Tapering opioid can be difficult and, for some patients, a very slow taper is most tolerable, e.g. 10% dose reduction monthly. If the patient has been treated with opioids for years, it may take over a year to taper to discontinuation. During this period, it will be helpful to have mental health support, and additional therapies in the comprehensive treatment plan roadmap actively incorporated: meditation, yoga, daily physical activity, group activities, distraction techniques, support animal if feasible, acupuncture, and other components can all be helpful.

In the second scenario, the patient has demonstrated side effects that are producing real or potential harms. In this situation, the patient needs to be tapered more rapidly so that safety is not compromised. The VA Opioid tapering tool available online provides useful information about pharmacological options that are available for managing many of the symptoms of withdrawal (Veterans Health Administration 2016). Prepare the patient for both acute and more persistent side effects of dose tapering: lacrimation, difficulty sleeping, anxiety, and restlessness are all transient and pass fairly quickly, body aches, tremor, and abdominal pains may persist for a few days with each dose reduction, whereas irritability, insomnia, fatigue, and increased body temperature may persist for longer periods. Schedule clinic visits more frequently during this tapering so that patient concerns and symptoms can be addressed. Anticipate that mental health support will need to be part of this process and that the elements of a solid comprehensive treatment plan will be necessary.

In the third scenario, a major threat to safety has occurred: either to the patient, the provider, or someone else – where there is a demonstrable relation to the prescription of opioids. An ultrarapid taper may be necessary. This can be highly unsettling for patients and substantive mental health stress may be present. Ensure that the patient has access to mental health support and that appropriate screening and assessment for suicidality is performed and support available. Opioids can be tapered as rapidly as 25% each day, close monitoring is appropriate and inpatient management

Table 49.1 Opioid WITHDRAWAL mnemonic – FLAPPY HANDS.

Fever and chills
Lacrimation
Agitation
Piloerection
Pupillary dilation
Yawning
--
Hypertension and tachychardia
Aches
Nausea
Diarrhea
Sweating

Table 49.2 Opioid OVERDOSE mnemonic – MORPHINE.

Myosis (pinpoint pupils)
Obtundation (sedation)
Respiratory suppression
Positive toxicology
Hypotension
Infrequency of output (constipation, urinary retention)
Nausea
Evidence of substance use disorder (injection sites, skin popping)

Pain Medicine at a Glance, First Edition. Beth B. Hogans.
© 2022 John Wiley & Sons Ltd. Published 2022 by John Wiley & Sons Ltd.

Table 49.3 Features of opioid tapering: paradigmatic scenarios.

Ultra-rapid taper	Rapid taper	Moderately slow taper
Patient, provider, caregiver, or others are at immediate risk	Patient is at risk of harm from opioids	Patient recognized opioids are not helping
Opioid withdrawal is not physiologically life-limiting but may provoke profound psychological distress and mild-severe physiological symptoms. Mental health access is important, patient may require assessment of emergent inpatient treatment	Opioid decreases may be associated with increased pain, patient may require increased resources, especially access to stable and qualified mental healthcare and nonpharmacological therapies, e.g. service animal, support groups	Opioid decreases may lead to pain exacerbation and mild anxiety, comprehensive pain therapies should be engaged to alleviate these subjective symptoms
Rate of dose decrease will be determined by maximally tolerated withdrawal effects and safety	Rate of dose decrease will be determined by dose-related harmful side effects that are not tolerable	Rate of dose decrease may be very slow, depending on nature of pain conditions and other comorbidities

Table 49.4 Naloxone – CDC-NIOSH recommendations.

Assess the incident scene
Call trained help (911)
Put on gloves and other PPE as needed
Evaluate (see mnemonic) for overdose
Administer naloxone intranasally or IM
According to formulation
Re-administer after 2–3 minutes
If no response to first dose
Render first aid until help arrives
Monitor, naloxone will wear off in minutes

may be appropriate and should be considered, according to local practice standards.

Whatever the pace, remember that opioid tapering is difficult for most patients. Take the opportunity to reflect aloud with the patient about the effort required, and whenever possible observe a moment of celebration and appreciation: ask the patient how they feel about what they have accomplished, and how they can safely celebrate a special milestone. Insight, appreciation, and trust are all important. Relapse may occur, but this should not cause the provider to change their therapeutic attitude toward the patient. Relapse can lead to life-threatening overdose and is serious. Nonetheless, giving the patient a sense that they are honored and valued as a person can increase the long-term prognosis for sustained recovery.

One of the critical challenges in tapering opioids is that sometimes people experience a serious pain flare and under certain circumstances they will be offered or may seek out in desperation, illicit opioids. This can be highly dangerous as doses are unregulated and inadvertent overdose may occur. With all patients receiving opioids, there should be a plan for overdose, i.e. naloxone (The National Institute for Occupational Safety and Health (NIOSH) hosted by CDC 2020) (Table 49.4). Naloxone is an opioid antagonist that is prescribed in the form of nasal spray in order to provide life-saving opioid-reversal in the event of opioid overdose. The risk of opioid overdose is compounded in patients tapering opioids as they will become less tolerant to high doses as the taper progresses.

References

Els, C., Jackson, T.D., Kunyk, D. et al. (2017). Adverse events associated with medium- and long-term use of opioids for chronic non-cancer pain: an overview of cochrane reviews. Cochrane Database of Systematic Reviews 10 (10): CD012509. https://doi.org/10.1002/14651858.CD012509.pub2.

The National Institute for Occupational Safety and Health (NIOSH) hosted by CDC (2020). Opioids in the Workplace: Responding to a suspected opioid overdose. https://www.cdc.gov/niosh/topics/opioids/response.html (accessed 13 August 2020).

Veterans Health Administration (2016). PBM Academic Detailing Service. Opioid Taper Decision Tool. https://www.pbm.va.gov/AcademicDetailingService/Documents/Pain_Opioid_Taper_Tool_IB_10_939_P96820.pdf (accessed 3 July 2020).

Pain in the young is characterized by several special features: (i) it can be heartbreaking, (ii) children may not have the ability to communicate verbally, (iii) young children will alter behavior without artifice to reduce pain, and (iv) most medications have not undergone rigorous testing in children, so that extra care is needed – most medication dosing is weight based.

At birth, the pain-sensing components of the nervous system are not completely myelinated. Myelination of the brain proceeds from front to back, it is widely appreciated that infants do not have especially clear vision for the first several months of life, and yet they can respond to familiar and appealing visual objects even before sharply focused vision occurs. By contrast, sound pathways are more reliably activated and responsive in normal neonates. The pain system is not fully activated in terms of cortical activity; nonetheless, there is much pain processing that occurs at the spinal and supraspinal (brainstem) levels, and this is important to know. The processing that occurs, even without involvement of the cortex, is dynamic, produces behavioral responses, and when exposed to strong activation, is sensitized to future stimuli – i.e., there is a reason we are acculturated to handling babies with care. One study examined infant males who underwent circumcision, with or without analgesia. The infants that did not receive analgesia at circumcision, cried more vigorously at the time of vaccination several weeks later, indicating measurable persistent change, suggestive of increased pain responsiveness.

Before the age of seven, infants, toddlers, and young children cannot be expected to reliably use the standard pain rating scales to communicate about pain. For this reason, behavioral pain scales have been developed and are used in an age-appropriate manner (University of Wisconsin Hospitals and Clinics Authority 2017) (Table 50.1). One scale for infants, the FLACC, assesses facial expression, movements, vocalization, and consolability (Figure 50.1). For verbal children, it may be appropriate to use a pictographic scale such as the FACES scale or the Wong–Baker scale. Sometime between 7 and 9, children develop the capacity to understand and use the numerical rating scale. Caregivers can also provide an assessment of pain and functional impacts of pain.

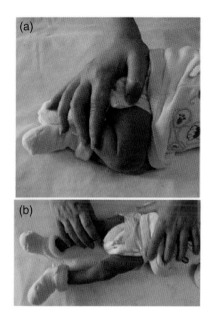

Figure 50.1 FLACC infant and small child pain scale. Source: Kucukoglu et al (2015). CC BY 4.0

Table 50.1 Neonatal/Infant pain scale. Source: Kucukoglu et al (2015). CC BY 4.0

Parameters	0 point	1 point	2 point
Facial expression	Relaxed	Grimace	-
Cry	No cry	Whimper	Vigorous crying
Breathing pattern	Relaxed	Change in breathing	-
Arms	Relaxed	Flexed/extended	-
Legs	Relaxed	Flexed/extended	-
State of Arousal	Sleeping/Awake	Fussy	-

Pain level: 0–2 points = No pain, 3–4 points = Moderate pain, >4 points = Severe pain

Table 50.2 Infant positioning for vaccination influences assessed pain. (a) Tucked position infants demonstrated fewer pain behaviors than (b) extended position infants (Data from Kucukoglu et al (2015)).

Categories	0	1	2
Face	No particular expression, or smile	Occasional grimace or frown, withdrawn, disinterested	Frequent to constant quivering chin, clenched jaw
Legs	Normal position, or relaxed	Uneasy, restless, tense	Kicking, or legs drawn up
Activity	Lying quietly, normal position, moves easily	Squirming, shifting back and forth, tense	Arched, rigid, or jerking
Cry	No cry (awake or asleep)	Moans or whimpers; occasional complaint	Crying steadily, screams or sobs, frequent complaints
Excitability	Content, relaxed	Reassured by occasional touching, hugging or being talked to, distractible	Difficult to console or comfort

When procedures are planned and performed, pain relief is very important for infants, children, and adolescents (Table 50.2). Recall that painful procedures are not a zero-sum game – pain experiences can and do result in changes to the nervous system that produce increased pain signaling in response to subsequent noxious

Table 50.3 Soothing and pain-relieving activities, by age group.

Neonate/Infant	Small child	Pre-adolescent	Teen
Holding gently while rocking	Holding gently while rocking	Holding or sitting next to	Attention to concerns
Swaddling (as instructed)	Tucking in, comfort pillows	Providing blankets/pillows	Providing physical needs
Repositioning	Repositioning, scene change	Repositioning, scene change	Change of scene, setting
Singing to or soft music	Singing to or soft music	Music or video, reading to	Music or video, reading with
Soothing touch, stroking	Soothing touch, stroking	Soothing touch, stroking	Access to friends
Comfort item: blanket, etc.	Comfort item: blanket, etc.	Engaging activity	Enjoyable activities

stimuli. Pain responses may be slightly delayed in younger children, but this does not mean they are not significant. As children age, the myelination of the brain and peripheral nerves increases and signaling occurs more quickly and precisely. Teenagers in particular have well-tuned pain-sensing abilities and despite appearing "all grown up" may have particular difficulty tolerating pain without support. One potential advantage is their capacity for intense absorption in videos so that distraction may be an especially useful nonpharmacological management option. Effective pain strategies vary according to age, but may include a range of options, combination of multiple non-invasive techniques may be utilized, e.g. distraction and topical EMLA cream prior to IV placement (Table 50.3).

Common pain-associated conditions in children include headache, musculoskeletal, pain related to developmental processes including skeletal-related pains, pain associated with accidents and trauma, pain related to infectious or inflammatory disease, e.g. ear infection, sore throat, toothache, and selected heritable conditions, e.g. sickle cell disease, familial migraine.

Migraine in one the most common pediatric pain-associated conditions. Presenting differently in young children, abdominal symptoms evolve into head pain around middle school age or puberty. Assessment for neurological deficits may be appropriate but unless clear deficits exist or a secondary headache syndrome is suspected, e.g. tumor, trauma, hemorrhage, infection, imaging is not appropriate (Hayes et al. 2018). Avoidance of triggers, including skipping meals, insufficient sleep, social stress, bright lights, loud noises is essential. Comprehensive pain management should be applied, counseling the parent or caregiver appropriately. Ibuprofen or acetaminophen can be utilized in weight-adjusted doses and is effective. Excessive or daily use must be avoided as transformed migraine or chronic daily headache may develop. Headache is generally prevalent in children, being present in about half of 7-year-olds and three-quarters of 15-year-olds.

Pediatric pain conditions include syndromes associated with growth and adaptation. In association with periods of mechanical stress shin splints, slipped capital femoral epiphysis, and low back pain may occur (Bernstein and Cozen 2007; Mahran et al. 2017; Taxter et al. 2014). Overuse syndromes including carpal tunnel syndrome, ulnar nerve compression, and lateral elbow tendinitis (tennis elbow) are not uncommon. Knee injuries are highly prevalent in young athletes and additional care is needed to provide adequate stretching and strengthening with special attention to knee and hip

muscles. Special attention should be paid to counseling adolescent patients and their parents regarding the life-long costs of inadequate rehabilitation – accelerated knee degeneration is a remarkably harmful state increasing risks for obesity, diabetes, and attendant conditions as the capacity for future physical activity is constrained.

Pain due to trauma and accidents is nearly universal in childhood. Instruction and guidance of parents in providing first aid analgesia, i.e. topical antiseptic with anesthetic (benzocaine) as well as rigorous wound care and tetanus vaccinations are essential. Fractures are often highly painful in children and analgesia should be provided according to local practice standards but without neglecting the child's needs for pain relief. Nonpharmacological measures can be actively incorporated during the daytime, e.g. video-distraction, cooling, engaging and fun activities, potentially allowing for oral analgesics at bedtime so that sleep is not disrupted by efforts at pain control.

References

Bernstein, R.M. and Cozen, H. (2007). Evaluation of back pain in children and adolescents. American Family Physician 76 (11): 1669–1676.

Hayes, L.L., Palasis, S. et al. (2018). Expert panel on pediatric imaging: ACR appropriateness criteria® headache-child. Journal of the American College of Radiology 15 (5S): S78–S90. https://doi.org/10.1016/j.jacr.2018.03.017.

Küçükoğlu, S., Kurt, S., and Aytekin, A. (2015). The effect of the facilitated tucking position in reducing vaccination-induced pain in newborns. Italian Journal of Pediatrics 41 (1): 61. https://doi.org/10.1186/s13052-015-0168-9. CC BY 4.0.

Mahran, M.A., Baraka, M.M., and Hefny, H.M. (2017). Slipped capital femoral epiphysis: a review of management in the hip impingement era. SICOT Journal 3: 35. https://doi.org/10.1051/sicotj/2017018. Epub 2017 May 17. PMID: 28513428; PMCID: PMC5434664.

Taxter, A.J., Chauvin, N.A., and Weiss, P.F. (2014). Diagnosis and treatment of low back pain in the pediatric population. The Physician and Sportsmedicine 42 (1): 94–104. https://doi.org/10.3810/psm.2014.02.2052. PMID: 24565826; PMCID: PMC4112374.

University of Wisconsin Hospitals and Clinics Authority (2017). Using pediatric pain scales. https://www.uwhealth.org/healthfacts/pain/7590.pdf (accessed 14 August 2020).

Pain is more prevalent in older adults than other populations. Painful musculoskeletal conditions increase with age; and 70% of older adults has one or more. Some argue that pain declines with age; recent data shows that pain increases with age until the tenth decade. Changes in pain processing with aging have mixed effects: declines in central pain-suppression mechanisms such as diffuse noxious inhibitory control (DNIC) and accumulating musculoskeletal changes increase pain; some pain pathway changes decrease pain even as many pain-coping mechanisms improve.

Low back pain (LBP) is the most prevalent pain in older adults; females have more LBP than males (Figure 51.1). LBP peaks around age 70–75 and remains high into the tenth decade. Older adults with LBP have low back conditions: spondylosis, sacroiliac dysfunction, stenosis, or facet osteoarthritis (OA). These conditions require comprehensive management – PT-directed exercise, ergonomic adjustments, moderate daily exercise, mindfulness, and meaningful activity. Swimming, water aerobics, dog walking, and chair yoga can all reduce LBP. Temporally, non-pharmacological therapies provide pain relief occurring over days to weeks – patients may need encouragement to stay the course. Especially when habituated to rapid relief from pills and injections, patients may by frustrated by the tempo of response.

Critically, healthcare providers must know the efficacy of non-pharmacological treatments. Recent meta-analysis provides details (Figure 25.1): the most effective therapies for chronic musculoskeletal conditions were Tai Chi and yoga. Sometimes patients resist adopting new therapies; Use the graph to show these treatments are as effective as medications. Injections may be appealing in selected circumstances but most commonly pain returns after a few weeks; pain injections are best understood as providing temporary relief so that rehabilitative therapies –especially PT – can occur. Pain injections almost always involve steroids, with negative side effects including diabetes, osteoporosis, skin thinning, muscle loss, and possible infections. Surgery may help specific patients but caution pertains with surgery for pain relief - chronic pain after surgery is not uncommon and rates increase with successive surgeries.

Osteoarthritis is extremely prevalent in older adults and comprehensive management is best (Figure 51.2). Importantly, focal pain signals arising from inflamed joints lead to reflexive muscle atrophy that is insidious and profound if unaddressed. Although biologically, this reflex provides pain relief – for an older adult, any muscle atrophy compounds age-related muscle loss (sarcopenia) leading to devastating weakness. For this reason, older adults must participate in physical therapy and daily exercise. Even in the patient anticipating joint replacement or joint injection, gentle and isometric exercises can prevent disastrous atrophy. Patients should understand the importance of limiting passive treatment therapies, e.g. pills, injections, surgeries, and value committing to active treatment approaches, including mindfulness, daily exercise, yoga/Tai Chi, ergonomics, sleep restoration, and PT. Dietary supplements may be beneficial but depend on the patient. Potential agents include turmeric, glucosamine chondroitin sulfate, probiotics, and vitamin D.

Diabetic peripheral neuropathy (DMPN) is prevalent in older adults; more common in men than women. Increased medical comorbidities characterize these patients: renal dysfunction, heart disease, hypertension, dyslipidemia; choosing treatments for these patients requires care. NSAIDs and acetaminophen have little benefit. Because DMPN pain is persistent, and opioids exhibit

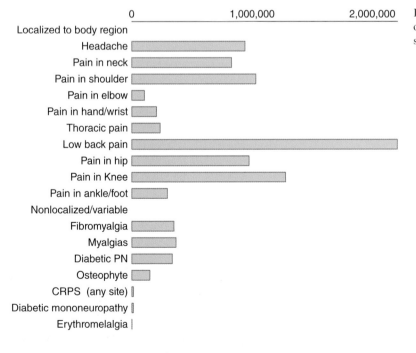

Figure 51.1 Common and less common pain conditions in older adults (total Medicare adults based on CMS 2017 data sample).

Pain Medicine at a Glance, First Edition. Beth B. Hogans.
© 2022 John Wiley & Sons Ltd. Published 2022 by John Wiley & Sons Ltd.

Figure 51.2 Adaptations to pain treatments for older adults.

Comprehensive older adult treatment: examples

Psychological support
Cognitive behavioral therapy
Mindfulness-based stress reduction
Acceptance-commitment therapy
Substance reduction/avoidance

Ergonomic adaptation
Cushioning and support
Footwear, cane, walker
Adaptive seating
Bathroom grab-bars

Mind-body
Gentle or seated yoga
Chi-gong vs. Tai Chi
Acupuncture/acupressure
Trigger points: neck, head, shoulders

Physical activity
Moderate daily exercise
Range of Motion
Gentle stretches

PAIN

Sleep
Sleep hygiene practices
Comfortable support

Passive strategies
(below the line)

'Safe standards'
Consider gastroprotection
for NSAIDs
Avoid daily use
Acetaminophen

**Interventions
(in reserve)**
Alternatives may pertain

Pain modulation
Consider topical agents
For oral agents: start low-go slow

tachyphylaxis (tolerance), DMPN and opioids are an undesirable combination. Pain-active antidepressants and gabapentinoids are preferred. Gabapentinoids can produce wooziness, and impair mental processing, positional cue processing, and cerebellar function, increasing falls. Falls are potentially life-altering, so gabapentinoids must "start low and go slow." Assess gait and sit-to-stand stability; prescribe a short course of PT for gait and balance. Comprehensive management includes moderate exercise, control of hyperglycemia, avoidance of dietary indiscretions, and blood sugar monitoring. DMPN patients benefit from comprehensive coordinated interprofessional care including primary care provider (PCP), podiatrist, PT, pharmacist, diabetes educator, and others including dieticians. Patients often ask about dietary supplements and diet: Alpha-lipoic acid may benefit both painful DMPN and diabetic cognitive dysfunction; vitamin B12 supplementation may be needed; vitamin D deficiency is associated with increased pain; and stringent avoidance of concentrated sweets is key. Finally, moderate daily activity and daily foot checks are necessary – several clinic visits are needed to optimize DMPN management.

Multimorbidity impacts the safety and choice of pain treatments (Booker and Herr 2020). Heart disease, renal failure, hypertension, and diabetes all shift the choices of pain medications and active treatments. Yoga can become chair yoga; Tai chi can become Qi gong (more gentle, flowing movements); a jog around the neighborhood becomes a 20-minute gentle stroll, Figure 51.3. Adapt the treatments to meet the patient where they are, even small gains are progress, and a new healthy habit is a step forward. Minimization of polypharmacy requires active inclusion of non-pharmacological therapies – group exercise programs can support both routine socialization and physical activity. Cognitive impairment can mean that patients need to make changes more slowly, despite this it is better for the healthcare provider to have a roadmap and know what the goals are: just as with smoking cessation, it is essential for doctors, nurses, and physician assistants to believe that smoking is harmful to health, so it is essential for healthcare providers to believe that non-pharmacological therapies are helpful and in aggregate create large positive changes. For metabolic effects of aging, see Chapter 52.

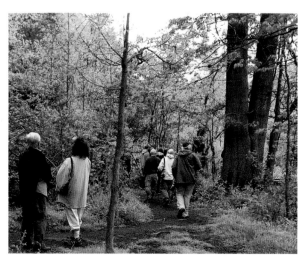

Figure 51.3 Bird-watching is an example of an activity that utilizes diverse skills that many older adults enjoy: gentle mobilization, observation, socializing, utilizing and sharing knowledge, and spending time outdoors. Volunteering, vocational activities, and hobbies are important sources of pleasure and meaning that can help reduce the impact of chronic pain. More moderately, vigorous activity may be required to activate endogenous pain-defense systems (endogenous analgesia); group exercise classes can be especially motivating for older adults.

The risks of pain in older adults are to some extent counterbalanced by the strengths of older adults in optimizing pain treatments. Often older adults can focus efforts on their own well-being. Older adults in many cases have strong psychological function and are quite emotionally resilient. Ally yourself with your patient and walk the journey with them, you will find older adults are remarkably engaged and positive in pursuit of patient-centered pain care.

Reference

Booker, S.Q. and Herr, K.A. (2020). Pain in older patients, chapter 19. In: *Pain Care Essentials* (eds. Hogans and Barreveld), 319–338. NY: Oxford University Press.

52 Tailoring pharmacotherapy in aging, renal, liver, and other metabolic dysfunctions

"Primum non nocere"

The famous dictum to first do no harm inspires many in the care of patients, for older adults and those with metabolic dysfunction, it is necessary to consider both patient and medication factors.

Aging imposes multiple changes on medication tolerability. Declines in lean muscle mass and increases adipose volumes (both central adipose accumulation and intramuscular fat) impact the pharmacokinetics of pain-active medications (Santanasto et al. 2017). Muscle relaxants and benzodiazepines persist for longer periods; long-acting clonazepam may be particularly hazardous.

Patient factors that impact medication choice include comorbidities, fall risks, and cognitive factors. Falls are a major concern: causing loss of independence in older adults – from hip, head, or spine trauma. Pain itself is associated with increased falls. Pain medications, including gabapentinoids, are associated with unsteadiness. Other factors include peripheral neuropathy, slowed mental processing, inner ear disease or vertigo, orthopedic conditions, and impaired vision or hearing. Cognitive impairment is another major risk for older adults receiving medications for pain – anticholinergic effects of antidepressants may be amplified. Gabapentinoids may cause confusion. Topiramate, which is used for chronic migraine, can at higher doses produce slowed cognition and impair word-finding. Patients may have specific susceptibilities to medication-associated side effects – GI bleeding, pulmonary dysfunction, vulnerability to cardiac electrophysiological effects, e.g. palpitations, conduction block; lower seizure threshold, or underlying renal or hepatic compromise.

Some medications have side effect profiles problematic for older adults. Opioids have profound effects at all levels of neurological functioning. Death is a real risk for vulnerable patients so that extreme caution is warranted. Opioids induce a depressed level of consciousness, together with decreased respiratory protection and respiratory drive (also from opioids), death may result. Tramadol, developed as a "safer alternative" to opioids, is a synthetic analgesic with both opioid- and benzodiazepine-like activity, so that similar concerns exist, along with a modest risk for seizures. Gabapentinoids, often correctly viewed as "safe" choices for neuropathic and persistent pain, have side effects that can be problematic for older adults with impaired balance or cognition. Falls, imbalance, unsteadiness, and wooziness, as well as impaired cognition, are all associated with gabapentinoids; these effects appear to be dose-related so that oftentimes the medications can still be used, but by introducing them at doses that are much lower than those prescribed for middle-aged or younger adults. With gabapentin for example – patients with impaired renal function or gait disturbance impacting balance, the medication should be started at a much reduced dose, e.g. 100 mg at bedtime, and tapered very slowly. Anticholinergic effects are common in patients treated with amitriptyline and other tricyclic anti-depressants – impairment leading to constipation, urinary retention, decreased sweating, and decreased saliva production each

with potential health harms. In addition, anticholinergic medications have impacts on cognitive functions and these include memory impairment, disorientation and confusion, difficulties with attention and concentration, and irritability (Lieberman 2004). All of the pain-active antidepressants have a black box warning for suicidality, and suicide risks remain high in older adults, second only to 45–64 year-olds group in suicide rates. Cardiac effects are also important in the tricyclic antidepressants and screening for baseline QTc prolongation with an EKG prior to initiating therapy is recommended for all those over age 40. Muscle relaxants produce confusion and sedation, which may be dangerous. Over-the-counter medications: NSAIDs are highly useful for the management of acute musculoskeletal pain but when used continuously, there is potential for harm from GI bleeding (Goldstein and Cryer 2015). Decrease NSAID amounts and duration to help prevent GI bleeding; and avoid altogether in those with GERD, Helicobacter pylori infection, peptic ulcer; or concomitant exposure to aspirin (ASA), anticoagulants, steroids, heavy tobacco or alcohol (Gwee et al. 2018). It is estimated that many thousand GI bleeding events occur annually due to NSAIDs; by contrast, acetaminophen-related deaths are much lower.

Renal failure is remarkably prevalent in older adults with moderate chronic renal disease diagnosed nearly 20% of older males and close to 15% of older females (Figure 52.1). Renal failure means that renal medication clearance is reduced and some medications must be avoided due to the potential for renal harm (Figure 52.2). In addition to decreased renal filtration and lower margin for tolerating nephrotoxicity, patients with renal failure very typically have anemia as the dysfunctional kidney produces less erythropoietin, essential for red cell production. Hypertension is present at very high rates in patients with renal failure. Taken together, these concurrent comorbidities make the use of NSAIDs harmful for patients with renal failure: whether due to excessive levels of NSAIDs, toxicity to the kidneys, the risks of GI bleeding

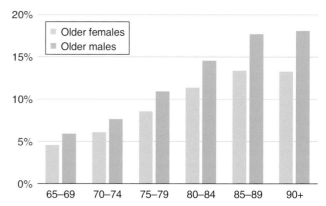

Figure 52.1 Moderate renal failure diagnosis increases with age, U.S. Medicare adults.

Pain Medicine at a Glance, First Edition. Beth B. Hogans.
© 2022 John Wiley & Sons Ltd. Published 2022 by John Wiley & Sons Ltd.

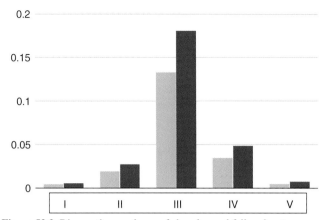

Figure 52.2 Diagnostic prevalence of chronic renal failure by stage, adults aged 90+.

in patients with anemia, or the increased rates of hypertensive and vascular occlusion events, e.g. heart attack or stroke (Figure 52.3). NSAIDs can also cause acute kidney injury in children as well as adults, and excessive NSAID use must be consistently avoided to prevent renal damage (Clavé et al. 2019).

Liver failure is less common than renal failure but also has implications for pain treatment selection. Acetaminophen should be limited in those with reduced liver function as fatal liver injury may occur and avoided altogether in those with hepatic impairment. NSAIDs may be used with caution, ibuprofen, is a "well-known but rare" cause of liver injury (LiverTox 2012). The tricyclic antidepressants have been associated with hepatotoxicity, by contrast the gabapentinoids are considered a safer choice. Several of the opioids demonstrate decreased metabolism with hepatic failure and dose adjustment and monitoring should follow local practice guidance.

Figure 52.3 Diagnostic prevalence of common conditions of older adults. Several of these conditions have important implications for treatment choice. The prevalence of hypertension and hyperlipidemia means that medications associated with increased risk of vascular events or hypertension would have increased risk. Conditions of diabetes, low back pain, and cataract indicate that falls risks are increased and medications that impair balance or delay CNS processing times will have increase potential for harm.

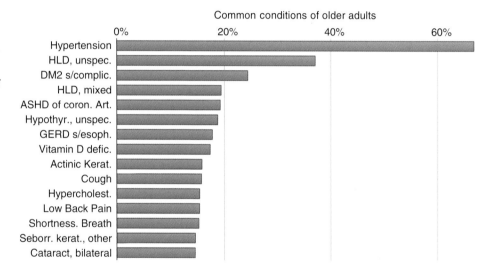

Nonpharmacological therapy should be included to reduce medication doses and harms, as well as improve functioning of the pain signaling system.

References

Clavé, S., Rousset-Rouvière, C., Daniel, L., and Tsimaratos, M. (2019). The invisible threat of non-steroidal anti-inflammatory drugs for kidneys. Front. Ped. 7: 520.

Goldstein, J.L. and Cryer, B. (2015). Gastrointestinal injury associated with NSAID use: a case study and review of risk factors and preventative strategies. Drug, Healthcare Pat. Saf. 7: 31–41.

Gwee, KA et al. (2018). Coprescribing proton-pump inhibitors with nonsteroidal anti-inflammatory drugs: risks versus benefits. J. Pain Res. 11: 361–74.

Lieberman, J.A. 3rd (2004). Managing anticholinergic side effects. The primary Care Companion to the Journal of Clinical Psychiatry 6 (Suppl 2): 20–23. Erratum in: Prim Care Companion J Clin Psychiatry. 2012;14(1):PCC.12lcx01362.

LiverTox (2012). Clinical and Research Information on Drug-Induced Liver Injury. Bethesda, MD: National Institute of Diabetes and Digestive and Kidney Diseases. Ibuprofen. (Updated 16 April 2018). https://www.ncbi.nlm.nih.gov/books/NBK547845/ (accessed 3 January 2021).

Santanasto, A.J., Goodpaster, B.H., Kritchevsky, S.B. et al. (2017). Body composition remodeling and mortality: the health aging and body composition study. J Geront. (A) 72:513–9.

Anatomy

The femoral and obturator nerves, as well as the lumbosacral plexus, pass through the pelvis and can be compressed in pregnancy, especially at the time of labor, but these syndromes remain uncommon. Carpal tunnel syndrome is increased during pregnancy, and this can manifest with hand or forearm pain.

Common and prevalent conditions

Headache is common in pregnancy, and severe headache may herald serious disease. Ominous headaches include severe headache of abrupt onset, in the most extreme form, this is referred to as "thunderclap" headache (Sharma et al. 2008). Eclampsia very often presents with severe headache; in fact, headache has been reported in almost 80% of women with preeclampsia (Ginzburg and Wolff 2009). Chest, epigastric, and right upper quadrant pain may all occur as symptoms of eclampsia. The sequelae of eclampsia may include death if not promptly recognized and treated. Additional signs and symptoms of eclampsia are noted in Table 53.1. Headache in pregnancy necessitates assessment, and elevation of blood pressure must be taken very seriously. The differential diagnosis of headache in the peripartum period is shown in Table 53.2. Obstetric and neurologic involvement are important. Once serious causes of pain are excluded, a comprehensive treatment approach, Figure 53.1, is especially useful in pregnancy; this will allow for avoidance of overreliance on medications, many of which are not appropriate during pregnancy, Figure 53.2.

Low back pain is very common in pregnancy and is best managed in most situations with an alternating regimen of short periods of rest alternating with periods of moderate physical activity as tolerated. Excessive stretching may be problematic during pregnancy as, as noted above, the body makes relaxins later in pregnancy, and these compounds may loosen ligaments so that unintentional dysfunction may occur. Therapies should be mindful of the pregnancy, e.g. pregnancy yoga. As noted above, the anterior, and posterior, joints of the pelvis may be prone to painful flares during later pregnancy. The round ligament is a source of sharp or stabbing pain, occurring commonly in the second trimester.

The **symphysis pubis** (anterior pelvic joint) is located at the center of the anterior pelvic rim, it can become acutely painful in mid-to-late pregnancy due to the release of "relaxins," compounds that cause a loosening of the normally stiff ligaments that bind the bones of the pelvic ring together. Pregnancy-related symphysis pubis pain can be severe and sharp, and curtail ambulation, but fortunately it often responds well to muscle-strengthening exercises focusing on the adductor muscles of the thigh. Analgesia should be avoided, although acetaminophen will be safe, it generally provides modest relief; PT can guide adductor muscle exercise, e.g. squeezing a ball between the knees, which can completely relieve pain; presupposing obstetrical and bladder issues have been excluded.

Pain management in pregnancy is consequential – changes in the coding system for drug use during pregnancy has made decision-making more complex. Acetaminophen is viewed as the safest choice in pregnancy, but the daily total amount of acetaminophen, from all sources, must be limited, and for those with liver impairment, amounts are more limited (FDA 2014; FDA 2015; LactMed 2018). Alcohol and acetaminophen should not be combined. NSAIDs are not recommended in the last trimester due to effects on the ductus arteriosus; some reports have concluded that there is increased risk of miscarriage in patients taking NSAIDs early in pregnancy, but FDA found these data were not conclusive (Koren et al. 2006; Drugs.com 2020; LactMed 2021a). Opioids have been potentially associated with neural tube defects, but CDC warns that opioid are associated with serious impacts on fetal development, as well as neonatal abstinence syndrome and sedation where opioids are taken during breastfeeding – they conclude that opioids should be avoided during pregnancy and breastfeeding (Purdue Pharma 2010; Yazdy et al. 2015; Lind et al. 2017; LactMed 2021b). The purpose of pain medication is to decrease the experience and implications of pain – these may include depression, anxiety, poor sleep, increased stress, and decreased cognitive function. Several of the medications utilized for management of chronic pain may not be ideal for use during pregnancy: anticonvulsants such as valproic acid, used for headaches, and carbamazepine, used for trigeminal neuralgia, are associated with neural tube defects. Duloxetine is

Table 53.1 Eclampsia: symptoms and signs.

Symptoms	Signs
Headache (severe, abrupt onset)	Hypertension
High blood pressure	Proteinuria
Ankle swelling	Increased reflexes
Epigastric pain	
RUQ pain	
Visual change	
Confusion	

Table 53.2 Peripartum headache differential diagnosis.

"Thunderclap" (sudden onset) – subarachnoid hemorrhage, preeclampsia/eclampsia, reversible cerebral vasoconstriction syndrome, cerebral venous thrombosis, low-pressure (dural-leak) headache
Constant or gradually worsening (non-thunderclap) – tension-type headache, cerebral vasculitis, transformed migraine, chronic daily headache, low-pressure (dural-leak) headache, medication withdrawal, migraine

Pain Medicine at a Glance, First Edition. Beth B. Hogans.
© 2022 John Wiley & Sons Ltd. Published 2022 by John Wiley & Sons Ltd.

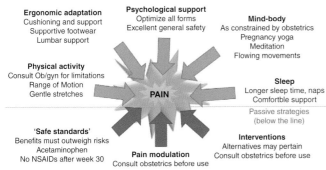

Figure 53.1 Comprehensive pain treatment planning for pregnancy and puerperium. Coordination of non-pharmacological therapies during pregnancy, delivery, and breastfeeding is extremely important. Pregnant mothers may be highly motivated to try non-medication therapies; and introducing cognitive behavioral therapy, acceptance commitment therapy, or mindfulness-based stress reduction may all set the stage for current and future success in comprehensive pain management.

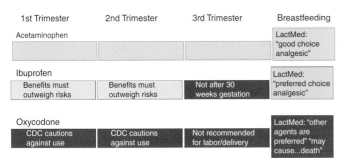

Figure 53.2 Graphic of basic analgesia medications, in pregnancy and breastfeeding: summary of selected medications and aggregated guidance from FDA, NIH, CDC, and reputable commercial information indicating cautions and warnings, see references.

unclassified for pregnancy, whereas gabapentin has previously been a Class C drug; studies have not indicated a strong risk for malformations or harm; however; more newborns were admitted to neonatal intensive care among those born to mothers treated with gabapentin (Fujii et al. 2013). Women should always consult their healthcare provider when taking or continuing to take pain medications during pregnancy.

Obstetrical pain control has radically transformed the birth experience for most women in high resource countries. Women can now "choose" to have a minimal pain birth, which most women prefer, or opt, in most cases, to approach the birthing process with a plan for natural childbirth. Given the uncertainties and the litigation-averse nature of the obstetrics profession, many physicians prefer their patients "chose to have an epidural." Those undergoing natural childbirth should know that if hormonal support, i.e. Pitocin, is needed for the labor, this will result in uterine contractions that are especially painful. In the event that an emergency C-section is required, the lack of an epidural in place may necessitate alternative approaches such as general anesthesia. Nonetheless,

the benefits of birth without an epidural include the satisfaction of a more natural birth experience; in some cases, the infant is more awake at birth, and less edema may be present. Advanced training and support by life partner and a doula or midwife may be especially beneficial. Attention to the control of pain in the perineum, after natural birth takes place, may include frequent ice packs and sitz baths.

References

Acetaminophen (2018). LactMed. https://www.ncbi.nlm.nih.gov/books/NBK501194/?report=reader (accessed 16 August 2020).

Drugs.com (2020). Ibuprofen pregnancy and breastfeeding warnings. https://www.drugs.com/pregnancy/ibuprofen.html (accessed 16 August 2020).

FDA (2014). Pregnant? Breastfeeding? Better drug information is coming. https://www.fda.gov/consumers/consumer-updates/pregnant-breastfeeding-better-drug-information-coming (accessed 16 August 2020).

FDA (2015). FDA has reviewed possible risks of pain medicine use during pregnancy; Safety Announcement. https://www.fda.gov/media/90209/download (accessed 10 May 2021).

Fujii, H., Goel, A., Bernard, N. et al. (2013). Pregnancy outcomes following gabapentin use: results of a prospective comparative cohort study. *Neurology* 80 (17): 1565–1570. https://doi.org/10.1212/WNL.0b013e31828f18c1.

Ginzburg, V.E. and Wolff, B. (2009). Headache and seizure on postpartum day 5: late postpartum eclampsia. *CMAJ* 180 (4): 425–428. https://doi.org/10.1503/cmaj.071446. PMID: 19221357; PMCID: PMC2638033.

Ibuprofen (2021a). LactMed. https://www.ncbi.nlm.nih.gov/books/NBK500986/?report=reader (accessed 16 August 2020).

Koren, G., Florescu, A., Moldovan Costei, A. et al. (2006). Nonsteroidal antiinflammatory drugs during third trimester and the risk of premature closure of the ductus arteriosus: a meta-analysis. *Annals of Pharmacotherapy* 40 (5): 824–829. [PubMed].

Lind, J.N., Interrante, J.D., Ailes, E.C. et al. (2017). Maternal use of opioids during pregnancy and congenital malformations: a systematic review. *Pediatrics* 139 (6): e20164131. https://doi.org/10.1542/peds.2016-4131.

Oxycodone (2021b). LactMed. https://www.ncbi.nlm.nih.gov/books/NBK501245/ (accessed 16 August 2020).

OXYCONTIN (2010). Oxycodone package insert. https://www.accessdata.fda.gov/drugsatfda_docs/label/2010/022272lbl.pdf (accessed 16 August 2020).

Sharma, P., Poppe, A.Y., Eesa, M. et al. (2008). Postpartum thunderclap headache. *CMAJ* 179 (10): 1033–1035. https://doi.org/10.1503/cmaj.080344.

Yazdy, M.M., Desai, R.J., and Brogly, S.B. (2015). Prescription opioids in pregnancy and birth outcomes: a review of the literature. *Journal of Pediatric Genetics* 4 (2): 56–70.

References

Dimitroulis, G. (2018). Management of temporomandibular joint disorders: a surgeon's perspective. Aust. Den. J. 63: S79–90.

Gauer, R.L. and Semidey, M.J. (2015). Diagnosis and treatment of temporomandibular disorders. Am. Fam. Phys. 91: 378–86.

Yoshiki I., et al. An updated review on pathophysiology and management of burning mouth syndrome with endocrinological, psychological and neuropathic perspectives. J Oral Rehabil. 46:574–87.

National Institute of Dental and Craniofacial Research (2020). Burning mouth syndrome. https://www.nidcr.nih.gov/sites/default/files/2017-12/burning-mouth-syndrome.pdf9 (acc. 6/9/20).

Sola, C., et al. (2020). Nerve blocks of the face, NYSORA (New York school of regional anesthesia). https://www.nysora.com/techniques/head- and-neck-blocks/nerve-blocks-face/ (accessed 9 June 2020).

Stuhr, S.H., et al (2014). Use of orthopedic manual physical therapy to manage chronic orofacial pain and tension-type headache in an adolescent. J Man Manip Ther. 22:51–8.

Dodds, KN et al. (2016). Glial contributions to visceral pain: implications for disease etiology and the female predominance of persistent pain. Transl. Psych. 6:e888.

Esophagitis. Mayo Clinic (2020). https://www.mayoclinic.org/diseases-conditions/esophagitis/symptoms-causes/syc-20361224 (acc. 8/13/20).

Kuhlmann, L et al. (2019). Patient and disease characteristics associate with sensory testing results in chronic pancreatitis. Clin. J. Pain 35:786–93.

Lee, IS et al (2019). Central and peripheral mechanism of acupuncture analgesia on visceral pain: a systematic review. Evid. Comp. Med. 2019: 1304152.

Mazzone, S.B. and Undem, B.J. (2016). Vagal afferent innervation of the airways in health and disease. Physiological Reviews 96:975–1024.

Meldgaard, T al. (2019). Pathophysiology and management of diabetic gastroenteropathy. Therapeutic Advances in Gastroenterology 12: 1756284819852047.

Moloney, RD et al (2015). Stress-induced visceral pain: toward animal models of irritable-bowel syndrome and associated comorbidities. Front. Psych. 6:15.

Olesen, AE et al. (2016). Management of chronic visceral pain. Pain Manag. 6:469–486.

Safdar, B. and D'Onofrio, G. (2016). Women and chest pain: recognizing the different faces of angina in the emergency department. Yale J Biol. Med. 89:227–38.

Singh, V.K. and Drewes, A.M. (2017). Medical management of pain in chronic pancreatitis. Dig. Dis. Sci. 62:1721–8.

Vila, AV et al. (2018). Gut microbiota composition and functional changes in inflammatory bowel disease and irritable bowel syndrome. Sci Transl Med 10 (472): eaap8914.

Yam, MF et al. (2018). General pathways of pain sensation and the major neurotransmitters involved in pain regulation. Intern. J Mol. Sci. 19:2164.

Cox, JJ et al. (2006). An SCN9A channelopathy causes congenital inability to experience pain. Nature 444:894–8.

Dib-Hajj, SD et al. (2005). Gain-of- function mutation in Nav1.7 in familial erythromelalgia induces bursting of sensory neurons. Brain 128: 1847–54.

Garvey, JF et al (2015). Epidemiological aspects of obstructive sleep apnea. J Thor. Dis. 7: 920–9.

Gracely RH et al (2002). Functional magnetic resonance imaging evidence of augmented pain processing in fibromyalgia. Arthr. Rheum. 46: 1333–43.

Kim, MK et al. (2013). Autonomic dysfunction in SCN9A-associated primary erythromelalgia. Clin. Auton. Res. 23: 105–7.

Marchettini, P et al. (2006). Painful peripheral neuropathies. Curr. Neuropharm. 4: 175–81.

Mease, PJ et al. (2009). The efficacy and safety of milnacipran for treatment of fibromyalgia. A randomized, double-blind, placebo-controlled trial. J. Rheum. 36:398–409.

Mezei, L et al. (2011). Pain education in North American medical schools. J. Pain 12:1199–1208.

Mitchell, S.W. (1872). Injuries of Nerves and Their Consequences. Philadelphia, PA: J.B. Lippincott.

Murinson, B.B. (2006). Painful neuropathy. In: Current Therapy in Neurological Disease (eds. J.W. Griffin, R.D. Johnson and J.C. McArthur). Mosby; Pages 363–8.

Murphy, K.R., Han, J.L., Yang, S. et al. (2017). Prevalence of specific types of pain diagnoses in a sample of United States adults. Pain Phys. 20:E257–68.

Petzke, F., Clauw, D.J., Ambrose, K. et al. (2003). Increased pain sensitivity in fibromyalgia: effects of stimulus type and mode of presentation. Pain 105:403–13.

Skelly, A.C., Chou, R., Dettori, J.R. et al. (2020). Noninvasive Nonpharmacological Treatment for Chronic Pain: A Systematic Review Update. Rockville (MD): Agency for Healthcare Research and Quality (US). Report No: 20-EHC009.

Wei, T al. (2009). Pentoxifylline attenuates nociceptive sensitization and cytokine expression in a tibia fracture rat model of complex regional pain syndrome. Eur. J. Pain 13 (3): 253–62.

Wolfe, F et al. (2010). The American College of Rheumatology preliminary diagnostic criteria for fibromyalgia and measurement of symptom severity. Arth. Care Res.62:600–10.

Murinson, B.B. (2011). Take Back Your Back. Beverly, MA: Fair Winds Press.

Vroomen, PC, et al. (1999). Lack of effectiveness of bed rest for sciatica. NEJM 340:418–23.

Wu, A , et al. (2020). Global low back pain prevalence and years lived with disability from 1990 to 2017. Ann Transl Med. 8:299.

Epstein, L.J. and Palmieri, M. (2012). Managing Chronic Pain With Spinal Cord Stimulation. Mount Sinai Journal of Medicine: A Journal of Translational and Personalized Medicine 79(1):123–32.

North, R.B. et al (2019). Redefining Spinal Cord Stimulation "Trials": A Randomized Controlled Trial Using Single-Stage Wireless Permanent Implantable Devices. Neuromodulation: Technology at the Neural Interface 23(1):96–101.

Garcia-Bonete, M.-J. et al (2019). A practical guide to developing virtual and augmented reality exercises for teaching structural biology. Biochem Mol Biol Educ, 47: 16–24.

General/Neuro/Pain brief exam (circle or tick findings)

Male Female Young Middle Older pleasant and cooperative

Mental status: Awake/alert
Orientation: date or   location or
Fund of knowledge: excel. v.good good fair poor
Speech: fluent dysarthric slurred paraphasic errors word finding
Naming: intact reduced parts naming: intact reduced absent
Repetition: intact or   crossed body: intact or

Cranial Nerves: PRRL ___ => ____ mm s/p cataract removal pinpoint dilated
EOMI; no nystagmus (R) fine coarse   (L) fine coarse INO IV VI
VFF to FC s ext.   (R) hemi quadr. (L) hemi quadr.
V1–V3 sensation to LT and sharp intact dec(R)   dec(L)
symmetrical grimace and eye closure (R)NLF (L)NLF (R)weak (L)weak
symmetrical hearing (R)dec. (L)dec. HOH
symmetrical u/p elevation (R)dn (L)dn symm. shoulder shrug
symmetrical tongue protrusion, movement is full tongue (R) (L)
neck flexion 5/5 and extension: 5/5 flex:___/5 ext:___/5

Motor: Bulk is normal   Tone is normal increased flaccid

	DEL	BIC	TRIC	WE	APB	FDI	ADV	IP	Quad	Hams	DF	PF	EHL
RT 5/5													
LT 5/5													

Pronator no (R)   (L)
Sensory: sharp testing present (B) UE and (B) LE   **hyperalgesia:**
proprioception 2mm 5mm 10mm absent
LT intact (B) UE (B) LE s/extinction c/extinction

Reflexes

Coordination:
F-t-N Intact (B)   fine tremor (L) (R)
Heel-shin: intact (B) dysmetric (R) (L)
Gait: normal slightly wide-based unsteady
        ataxic weak:_____ not tested
Toe-gait: nl unsteady heel-gait: nl unsteady
Tandem: nl unsteady Station normal forward
Stands eyes closed well unsteady

Tenderness to palpation (moderate or greater)
(R) scalp cervical thoracic lumbar paraspinals
        SI joint piriformis m. hip knee ankle other:
(L) scalp cervical thoracic lumbar paraspinals
        SI joint piriformis m. hip knee ankle other:

Range of motion (normal, without pain)
(R) shoulder wrist SLR (straight leg raise) hip knee other:
(L) shoulder wrist SLR (straight leg raise) hip knee other:
Neck flexion extension R turning L turning R bend L bend
Back flexion extension R turning L turning R bend L bend

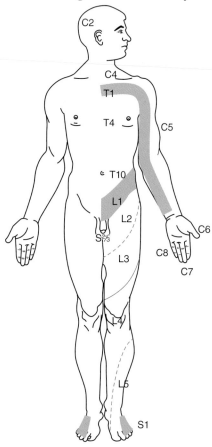

Pain diagram/dermatome key.

Developed by BBH from Public domain material (Gray's Anatomy, 1918); dermatomes aggregated from Duus, O'Brien, Netter, AccessAnesthesiology.

Pain Medicine at a Glance, First Edition. Beth B. Hogans.
© 2022 John Wiley & Sons Ltd. Published 2022 by John Wiley & Sons Ltd.

Appendix II: Sample pain diary worksheet

PAIN DIARY WORKSHEET   **Month:** _____

Sunday	Monday	Tuesday	Wednesday	Thursday	Friday	Saturday

Pain problems: A – _____ B – _____ C – _____

Instructions for the pain diary:

Each day, record your pain intensity on a scale from 0 (no pain) to 10 (worst pain imaginable).

If you have more than one pain type, e.g. migraine headache, tension headache, and knee pain, you can use a letter or color code to indicate which pain you are recording and how long the problem was present on a specific day. For example, you could put: "A–7, three hours" to indicate that for problem "A" (migraine headache in this example) you had pain of 7 out of 10 severity for three hours.

You should also note any changes in medications, or unusual activities.

Example of completed diary for two weeks:

Sunday	Monday	Tuesday	Wednesday	Thursday	Friday	Saturday
A–7, three hours			A–6, eight hours	A–9, two hours triptan		
	B–5, four hours ibuprofen				One glass of red wine	
Hiking	C–4, six hours Icepack	C–3, four hours Icepack		B–4, three hours Acetamin		Two cocktails

Pain types: A: "migraine," B: "tension headache," C: left knee pain.

Pain Medicine at a Glance, First Edition. Beth B. Hogans.
© 2022 John Wiley & Sons Ltd. Published 2022 by John Wiley & Sons Ltd.

Abuse: A term employed in the prior version of the Diagnostic and Statistical Manual of Mental Disorders (DSM-IV) to indicate a milder form of substance use disorder. This term remains in current use due to integration into the presently utilized version of the International Classification of Disorders (ICD-10) adapted for use in the United States.

Addiction: Not formally defined as a mental disorder, addiction is defined by the National Institute of Drug Abuse as a severe relapsing condition with "compulsive drug seeking despite negative consequences." The 6 C's are often used as an aid to recalling the pertinent features: a Chronic, Condition (of the brain), featuring Compulsive, Continued use, despite Consequences, with a lack of Concern for associated harms. The term was replaced by the terms "abuse" and "dependence" with a prior diagnostic revision and more recently by the term "substance use disorder" rated in terms of severity (mild, moderate, severe).[1]

Allodynia: pain in response to a normally nonpainful stimulus, intense pain when exposing steam-burned skin to warm water.

Analgesic: A substance that relieves pain. At present, all of the widely available analgesic agents have the potential for serious harms, e.g. NSAIDs can cause life-threating gastrointestinal bleeding, opioids can cause life-threatening respiratory suppression.

Anesthetic: A substance that induces insensitivity to pain. Many of these compounds cannot be used for ordinary pain control due to profound side effects, an example of this is lidocaine which can cause life-threatening cardiac arrythmias.

Central sensitization: a process of increasing responsiveness of central nervous system pathways that results in increased pain for patients with that pain being more difficult to treat and slower to resolve.

Dependence: A term employed in the prior version of the Diagnostic and Statistical Manual of Mental Disorders (DSM-IV) to indicate a more severe form of substance use disorder. This term remains in current use due to integration into the presently utilized version of the International Classification of Disorders (ICD-10) adapted for use in the United States. In a mechanism-focused context, dependence takes the form of physical or psychological dependence. There are profound changes in the brain and body in response to exposure to stimuli, including drugs, that activate the reward pathway. Physical dependence is defined by the presence of physical withdrawal symptoms, such as tremor, diarrhea, or lacrimation, upon withdrawal of the stimulus, e.g. morphine, heroin, and cocaine. Physiological dependence is defined by the presence of psychological symptoms, such as anxiety, depression, paranoia, upon withdrawal of the stimulus.

Dorsal column: Heavily myelinated vertical section of the spinal cord, situated posteriorly (dorsal aspect), and serving as a conduit for large sensory fibers subserving vibration and position sense.

Stimulation of these structures may impede pain signaling, a phenomenon utilized in some forms of pain treatment.

Hyperalgesia: increased pain in response to a normally painful stimulus, i.e., extreme pain in response to a pinprick.[2]

Misuse: NIDA uses this term essentially synonymously with abuse[1]

Narcotic: an antiquated term previously used to refer to a group of medications with sedative properties.[3] The term is cemented in drug terminology by use in entitling the foundational U.S. federal legislation regulating opioids and other drugs in 1914 and ensuing use as a term of reference to drugs subject to legal control.[4]

Opiate: substances made from opium or containing opium. The preferrable term is opioid which includes a larger range of relevant substances.[5]

Opioids: substances resembling or consisting of opium and related compounds. Prescription opioids are, per the Food and Drug Administration (FDA), "powerful pain-relieving medications" associated with serious potential harms, such as addiction.[6]

Pain: The word pain is used widely in the English language to indicate "unpleasant experiences" in a wide range of settings ranging from economic events, e.g., "Investor pain following stock marked adjustment" to teenage heartache. We refrain from referring to pain in the medical context as "physical pain" because pain has many impacts on the body and brain, including mental and emotional impacts so that even "purely nociceptive pain" has profound impacts on the person that extend beyond the "physical." The IASP has recently revised their definition of pain, the new definition is: "An unpleasant sensory and emotional experience associated with, or resembling that associated with, actual or potential tissue damage."[2]

Peripheral nerve: Structures in the peripheral nervous system serving as conduits for axons connecting peripheral afferent nerve terminals to the dorsal root ganglia (DRGs) wherein reside the primary sensory neurons. Between the DRGs and the dorsal root entry zone in the dorsal spinal cord, the conduit structure is the sensory nerve root. Compression of this nerve root is referred to "radiculopathy," a term originating from the Latin term radicula for "little root."

Substance Use Disorder: A DSM-based diagnosis of disordered substance use that includes impaired control, e.g., taking larger than intended quantities; social impairment, e.g. recurrent interpersonal problems; risky use; and pharmacological criteria, i.e., tolerance and withdrawal. Graded as mild, moderate, or severe according to specified criteria.[7]

Substantia gelatinosa: Superficial layers of the spinal dorsal horn neurons, i.e., Rexed laminae I and II, involved in nociceptive signaling.

Pain Medicine at a Glance, First Edition. Beth B. Hogans.
© 2022 John Wiley & Sons Ltd. Published 2022 by John Wiley & Sons Ltd.

Sources

1. https://www.drugabuse.gov/publications/media-guide/science-drug-use-addiction-basics

2. https://www.iasp-pain.org/terminology?navItemNumber=576#Multimodaltreatment

3. https://www.dea.gov/taxonomy/term/331

4. https://govtrackus.s3.amazonaws.com/legislink/pdf/stat/38/STATUTE-38-Pg785.pdf

5. https://www.cancer.gov/publications/dictionaries/cancer-terms/def/opiate

6. https://www.fda.gov/drugs/information-drug-class/opioid-medications

7. https://www.ncbi.nlm.nih.gov/books/NBK92053/table/ch2.t5

Consult your physical therapist for details on performing these activities and for additional, specific recommendations

- Chin tucks: stretch and strengthen cervical muscles – retract chin towards the center of the neck
- Ear-to-shoulder: stretch and strengthen lateral strap muscles of the neck – lateral flexion to either side
- Scapular retraction: improve posture and reduce mid-back pain – contract rhomboid muscles
- Shoulder circles: prevent frozen shoulder and avoid chronic shoulder pain – 10 circles each side daily
- Upper limb nerve glides: multiple flexion-extension motions designed to stretch and release pressure on nerves
- Pelvic tilts: stretch lower spine and strengthen abdominal muscles building spinal support
- Knee-to-shoulder: release hip and buttock muscles – prevent piriformis syndrome and sciatica
- Knee-to-opposite-shoulder: deeper release of piriformis and gemelli muscles of buttock – sciatica prevention
- Lower limb nerve glides: seated knee extension movements repeated to prevent sciatic nerve compression

- Iliopsoas stretch: Standing lunge (may begin gently) to prevent contraction of deep anterior hip muscles
- Hamstring stretch: Lying or standing depending on SI joint stability – prevent weakening of key thigh muscles
- Glut strengthening: Walking sideways in knees-bent position, may use ankle-bands to increase effort – essential exercise to maintain gait stability in aging
- Ankle dips: With support for balance, stand with toes on exercise step, dip heels low and then rise onto toes – key ankle strengthening exercise important for stable gait
- Toe lifts: while holding a secure object for balance, raise toes into air while balancing on heels – builds tibialis anterior strength important for secure walking (clearing objects with toe)
- One-legged stands: while holding a secure object for balance, practice standing on one foot for up to a minute, make this more challenging by standing on foam or a balance-disc, target 60 seconds – helps build strength and proprioceptive awareness.

Comprehensive, coordinated pain self-management

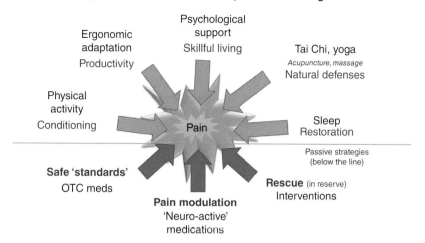

Given it is not healthy for anyone to rely only on painkillers long-term, I would be interested in trying the following:

Physical Therapy	Yoga	Acupuncture
Occupational therapy	Daily walks	Massage
Dance	Ice	Self-massage
Art	Heat packs	TENS
Music	Heating pad	Sleep clinic
Meditation	Psychology	Ergonomics
Talk therapy	Tai Chi	Dietary changes

Risks of treatment that are too intense for me to accept:

_____

Side effects that I cannot tolerate: _____

Side effects that I don't like: _____

Costs of treatment that currently prevent me from getting better:

_____

Barriers that currently interfere with me getting better: _____

_____

Bio – Psycho – Social Model
(many factors contribute to chronic pain)
Circle all that apply – discuss with your doctor or PCP

Biological	Psychological	Social
Disc/joint/bone degeneration	Depression	Smoking
	Anxiety	Poor ergonomics
Facet joint arthritis	PTSD	Lack of exercise
Ingrowth of pain-type nerve endings	Post-TBI	Stress
	Other mental illness	Physical demands
Ligamentous stretch or hypertrophy	Dysphoria	Poor sleep
	Somatic focus	De-conditioning
Muscle strain	Low self-efficacy	Lack of social suppor
Radiculopathy	Substance abuse	
Altered central pain processing	Personality d/o	Expectations

Three things I would like to do if pain was not 'holding me back':
1) _____
2) _____
3) _____

Three things that I really value in life (people, ideas, things, activities)
1) _____
2) _____
3) _____

My confidence that I can overcome pain (rate from 0 to 10): _____
My commitment to overcoming pain (rate from 0 to 10): _____

Multiple choice questions

Chapter 1 – Pain: what it is and how we begin to assess it

1. **The following are correct about pain:**
   a. Pain is not well understood
   b. Pain is not important in a clinical setting
   c. Pain is something that patients must endure
   d. Pain is a sensory and emotional experience
   e. Pain has little impact on clinical outcomes
2. **The following are correct about standard biomedical (mechanism-focused) assessment of pain except:**
   a. It includes the quality of pain
   b. It includes the region affected by pain
   c. It includes the severity of the pain
   d. It includes the impact of pain on work performance
   e. It includes the timing of pain
3. **The following are correct about functional pain assessment except:**
   a. It includes the impact of pain duration
   b. It includes impact of pain on sleep
   c. It includes impact of pain on friendships
   d. It includes impact of pain on self-care
   e. It includes impact of pain on capacity to carry out ordinary tasks at work or school

Chapter 2 – Nociceptive processing: How does pain occur?

1. **Nociceptive processing refers to:**
   a. The processing of nociceptins by the immune system
   b. The processing of pain signals by the nervous system
   c. The binding of nociceptikines by receptor molecules
   d. The activation of the cortical pain center in the frontal lobe
2. **Nociceptive processing system includes the following components except:**
   a. Transmission
   b. Transduction
   c. Induction
   d. Perception
   e. Modulation
3. **The following structures are involved in the transmission of pain except:**
   a. Primary afferent peripheral nerve terminal
   b. Primary afferent central terminal
   c. Spinal cord
   d. Thalamus
   e. Dorsal root ganglion

Chapter 3 – What are the major types of pain?

1. **The following are correct regarding nociceptive pain except:**
   a. Nociceptive pain is highly responsive to treatment
   b. Nociceptive pain is associated with responses to trauma
   c. Nociceptive pain typically results in long-lasting changes to the nervous system that lead to permanent pain` sensitivity
   d. Nociceptive pain involves mediator signals related to cell injury such as bradykinin and protons
   e. Nociceptive pain is unpleasant and associated with suffering when untreated
2. **Inflammatory pain is characterized by all the following except:**
   a. Heightened sensitivity to stimuli that are normally not painful
   b. Poor response to short-term opioids
   c. Overall good response to NSAIDs
   d. Is associated with pain related to abscess, sunburn, and osteoarthritis
   e. Can co-occur with other pain mechanisms, e.g. nociceptive, neuropathic
3. **The following are correct regarding neuropathic pain, except:**
   a. Poorly responsive to NSAIDs
   b. Overall good response to long-term opioids
   c. Associated with conditions such as diabetic neuropathy, radiculopathy
   d. Characterized by unusual sensations such as zinging, tingling, and electric shocks
   e. Potentially responsive to neuromodulating medications such as pain-active antidepressants and pain-active anticonvulsants

Chapter 4 – How prevalent is pain and what are the common forms?

1. **Which of the following is incorrect regarding the prevalence of pain:**
   a. Untreated cancer pain is estimated to affect 4.8 million people
   b. Availability of opioids for pain relief varies by two orders of magnitude between high-resource and low-resource countries

c. Fibromyalgia is the most prevalent cause of chronic pain worldwide

d. Low back pain is the most prevalent cause of work-related disability in the United States

2. **Which of the following is correct regarding the gender differences in pain:**
   a. All men can tolerate more pain than women
   b. Most men experience relatively little pain
   c. Pain medications do not work as well for women
   d. Differences between how men and women experience pain are real but subtle

3. **The following statements about pain treatments are correct except:**
   a. Opioids are highly effective for nociceptive pain and widely used
   b. The rate of drug overdose deaths has increased with opioid prescribing
   c. Efficient safeguards are in place to prevent opioid abuse
   d. Non-pharmacological treatments for pain are not widely used but have the potential to reduce over-reliance on opioids

Chapter 5 – Pain and ethical practice: How do we resolve dilemmas in pain care?

1. **The "Four Pillars of medical ethics" include the following except:**
   a. Beneficence
   b. Advocacy
   c. Non-maleficence
   d. Distributive justice
   e. Autonomy

2. **In pain care, beneficence means the following except:**
   a. Seeking to provide pain relief
   b. Endeavoring to improve a patient's level of function
   c. Placing the patient's comfort ahead of other concerns
   d. Taking steps to limit adverse effects of pain treatments

3. **In addition to the four pillars of medical ethics, the practice of pain care is guided by the following except:**
   a. Relevant codes of ethics
   b. Ideals including compassion and interpersonal awareness
   c. A capacity for self-regulation and resilience
   d. Self-indulgence and self-assuredness
   e. An insightful awareness of one's professional limitations

Chapter 6 – Advanced skillfulness in clinical practice: the big challenges

1. **All of the following can present big challenges to pain medicine except:**
   a. Patients not exhibiting curiosity about non-pharmacological treatments

b. Determining the origin of pain in some patients

c. Interpreting a patient's description of what their pain feels like

d. Understanding why a pain problem keeps recurring even when treated

2. **The following are examples of pain referral patterns, except:**
   a. Viscerotomes
   b. Coliotomes
   c. Myotomes
   d. Sclerotomes
   e. Dermatomes

3. **The following correctly match the referred pain pattern to the pain-producing structure except:**
   a. Viscerotomes: viscera
   b. Sclerotomes: bone
   c. Myotomes: muscle
   d. Dermatomes: skin

Chapter 7 – Cognitive factors that influence pain

1. **Which of the following cognitive phenomena has the capacity to decrease pain:**
   a. Catastrophizing about the pain problem
   b. Anxiety
   c. Social exclusion by a stranger
   d. Distraction, e.g. a video game

2. **Which of the following is an example of a statement by a patient indicating positive self-efficacy:**
   a. "I believe that only you can fix me doc."
   b. "I feel a lot better with those tablets."
   c. "I think if I start exercising, I will feel better."
   d. "My family is really supportive of my recovery."

3. **All of the following are examples of catastrophizing except:**
   a. Rumination
   b. Absorption
   c. Magnification
   d. Helplessness

Chapter 8 – Approach to the patient with pain: conceptual models of care and related terminology

1. **All of the following are basic processes included in the mechanisms-based classification of pain except:**
   a. Nociceptive
   b. Oncologic
   c. Neuropathic
   d. Inflammatory

2. **The following are examples of disease-centered approach to pain medicine, except:**
   a. Patient has severe pain in response to a torn ligament, resolution is expected to be protracted

b. Patient has severe pain in response to a muscle pull, resolution is expected to be rapid

c. Patient has severe pain in response to a migraine, rapid resolution is expected to depend on prompt administration of medication

d. Patient has severe pain in response to a minor fall, no specific cause of the pain has been identified, resolution in response to OTC analgesia is expected

e. Patient has severe pain in response to peripheral neuropathy, resolution is expected to be very protracted

3. **The following choices correctly match the expected affective response to clinical context except:**

a. Being told that nothing more can be done to resolve a pain-associated condition: dismay

b. Suffering chronic pain as the result of medical mishap: suspicion

c. Undergoing a demanding physical examination: stress

d. Conveying your medical history to a new healthcare provider for the 21st time: enthusiasm

e. Finding a healthcare provider who uses active listening and follows through on commitments to help: relief

Chapter 9 – The pain-focused clinical history: well-developed illness narratives impact pain outcomes

1. **Asking open-ended questions will encourage the following except:**

a. The patient in providing a pain-focused illness narrative

b. The clinician in identifying the cardinal features of a pain-associated condition, e.g. timing, location

c. The development of an therapeutic alliance

d. The fostering of biases that interfere with rapport building

e. Lead the clinician toward insight into the patient's health-related values and function

2. **The cardinal features of pain include the following except:**

a. Quality

b. Region

c. Sensitivity

d. Timing

e. Usually associated (with) findings

3. **Which of the following statement is not correct**

a. The biomedical model of pain addresses the physiological and pathological factors that lead to pain

b. The biomedical model of pain includes identifying a pain generator

c. The biopsychosocial model includes an assessment of psychological impacts, e.g. anxiety related to pain

d. The biopsychosocial model considers factors such as work or learning-related dysfunction that may amplify pain

e. The biopsychosocial model of pain explicitly excludes identifying pathology causing the pain

Chapter 10 – Assessing pain in those with communication barriers

1. **The following are correct about pain:**

a. Pain cannot be assessed in nonverbal patients

b. Pain is difficult for patients to understand

c. Pain assessment can be capably performed using different approaches

2. **The following is incorrect about communication barriers to pain assessment:**

a. A patient with dysarthria may not be able to use a pain scale

b. A patient with expressive aphasia may not be able to use a pain scale

c. A patient with receptive aphasia may not be able to use a pain scale

d. A patient with hearing impairment may be able to use a pain scale

3. **The following are correct about behavioral pain assessment except:**

a. It is appropriate for patients with advanced dementia

b. It is appropriate for infants

c. It is appropriate for small children

d. It is appropriate for patients without communication barriers

Chapter 11 – Examination skills I: interaction, observation, and affect

1. **Guarding, wincing, and vocalization are pain behaviors most characteristic of the:**

a. Hyperacute phase of pain

b. Acute phase of pain

c. Chronic phase of pain

d. None of the above

2. **All of the following are elements of the NURSE acronym for management of affect in the clinical encounter except:**

a. Name

b. Understand

c. Respect

d. Support

e. Evaluate

3. **Behaviors that support the development of trust and rapport include:**

a. Sitting at eye level with the patient during the history-gathering process

b. Having open body language, e.g. facing the patient with legs and arms uncrossed

c. Leaning slightly forward

d. Documenting all comments verbatim using a recording device

e. Maintaining a neutral facial expression, with mild expressions of concern or support

Chapter 12 – Examination skills II: inspection and manual skills

1. **Testing of biceps for strength evaluates activation of the following nerve roots:**
   a. C5–6
   b. C6–7
   c. C7–8
   d. C8/T1

2. **Which reflex is depressed with L5 nerve root compression?**
   a. Patellar
   b. Ankle jerk
   c. Plantar response
   d. None of the above

3. **The following are appropriate for the testing of sharp sensation except**
   a. A standard safety pin
   b. The broken end of a cotton tip applicator
   c. A proprietary neuro-testing tip

Chapter 13 – Integrating knowledge, skills, and compassionate practices

1. **The following are domains of clinical competence as defined by Epstein and Hundert except:**
   a. Knowledge
   b. Emotion
   c. Reflection
   d. Values
   e. Supervisory capacity

2. **The following are dimensions of emotional competence as described here, except:**
   a. Emotional strength
   b. Emotional flexibility
   c. Emotional resilience
   d. Emotional regulation
   e. Emotional intelligence

3. **The following are part of how students are evaluated against standards in clinical care:**
   a. Subjective assessment
   b. Clinical competencies
   c. Competitive comparison
   d. Practice performance
   e. Observation checklists

Chapter 14 – Motivational interviewing and shared decision-making: psychological skills in primary care for pain

1. **Which of the following does not represent a correct pairing of stage in "stages of change" model and cognitive activity?**
   a. Precontemplative: maintaining behavior
   b. Contemplative: weighing costs of change
   c. Preparation: experimenting with change
   d. Action: taking steps to change
   e. Relapse: feels demoralization

2. **Techniques to support the person in relapse include:**
   a. Expressing empathy
   b. Developing discrepancies
   c. Resisting resistance
   d. Supporting self-efficacy
   e. Tough talk

3. **Emanuel and Emanuel famously described patients as varying in terms of autonomy in healthcare decision-making; in addition, when making health-related decisions, patients may constructively be thought of as having varying:**
   a. Health-related knowledge
   b. Health-related values
   c. Health-related discernment

Chapter 15 – Communicating with teams caring for patients with pain

1. **Landmark Joint Commission foundational standards on pain included the following:**
   a. The hospital educates all licensed independent practitioners about assessing and managing pain
   b. The hospital educates fully employed practitioners about assessing and managing pain
   c. The hospital educates all licensed independent practitioners about referring patients for pain management
   d. The hospital educates fully employed practitioners about referring patients for pain management

2. **The following strategies are useful for acute pain care management except:**
   a. Observational pain scales in awake, verbal adults
   b. Pain plan-of-care checklist
   c. Coordination of pharmacological and non-pharmacological treatments
   d. Protocol for reporting inadequate pain relief and side effects
   e. In-service education about pain

3. **Chronic opioid exposure can challenge teams providing care for patients with complex pain conditions through the following mechanisms except:**
   a. Normal enhancement to opioid analgesia over time in patients with chronic opioid exposure
   b. Increased pain sensitivity in patients with chronic opioid exposure
   c. Decreased pain tolerance in patients with chronic opioid exposure
   d. Decreased pain thresholds in patients with chronic opioid exposure

Chapter 16 – Planning therapy: coordinated, comprehensive, patient-centered care

1. **The following are elements of a comprehensive pain management plan except:**
   a. Sleep optimization
   b. Physical therapy or HEP
   c. Meditation and/or relaxation
   d. OTC medications
   e. Opioids to the exclusion of other medications

2. **The following are important determinants of what is ultimately included in comprehensive pain management plan except:**
   a. Patient preference
   b. Costs of time and money
   c. Evidence for efficacy
   d. Referral incentive plans
   e. Long-term impact on patient health

3. **The following pairs correctly identify passive and active pain management strategies except:**
   a. Injection of medication by pain interventionalist: active
   b. Taking OTC medication correctly: passive
   c. Yoga lessons: active
   d. Meditation practice: active
   e. Developing new healthy sleep habits: active

Chapter 17 – Basic considerations for pharmacological therapy – balancing mechanisms of drugs and disease

1. **Identify which of the mechanism: medication class pairings is not correct:**
   a. Mild nociceptive pain: over-the-counter analgesia
   b. Moderate-to-severe nociceptive pain: prescription combination analgesia, i.e. Percocet
   c. Moderate inflammatory pain: NSAIDs
   d. Moderate neuropathic pain: NSAIDs
   e. Mild neuropathic pain: low-dose neuromodulating agents

2. **Which of the following conditions is likely to have multiple basic pain mechanisms and potentially require the use of multiple pain-active medications**
   a. Herpes zoster
   b. Myocardial infarction
   c. Dental extraction
   d. Low back pain
   e. Simple laceration

3. **All of the following are important for reducing potential adverse effects of medications except:**
   a. Making sure the patient is aware of potential adverse effects
   b. Avoiding shared decision-making in the treatment of pain patients
   c. Screening for known risks such as potential for opioid abuse
   d. Obtaining monitoring blood work in patients treated with some anticonvulsants

Chapter 18 – Nonsteroidal anti-inflammatory drugs (NSAIDs) and acetaminophen (over-the-counter analgesia)

1. **NSAIDs are valuable as a result of the following except:**
   a. Potency against mild-to-moderate nociceptive pain
   b. Potency against mild-to-moderate inflammatory pain
   c. Potency against mild-to-moderate neuropathic pain

2. **NSAIDs are contraindicated for the following patients except:**
   a. Advanced renal failure
   b. History of recurrent GI bleeding
   c. Patients in the third trimester of pregnancy
   d. Patients with mild liver failure
   e. Patients with a history of NSAID-induced anaphylaxis

3. **Acetaminophen should be avoided in the following types of patients except:**
   a. Active alcohol abuse
   b. Third trimester of pregnancy
   c. Liver failure
   d. Patients taking multiple Percocets daily

Chapter 19 – Neuromodulating agents: pain-active antidepressants and anticonvulsants

1. **Neuromodulating agents for the treatment of neuropathic pain include the following medication classes:**
   a. Over-the-counter analgesics
   b. Selective serotonin reuptake inhibitors (antidepressants)
   c. Selected anticonvulsants
   d. Opioids

2. **Pain-active antidepressants include the following except:**
   a. Fluoxetine
   b. Duloxetine
   c. Amitriptyline
   d. Venlafaxine
   e. Nortriptyline

3. **Pain-active anticonvulsants include the following except:**
   a. Carbamazepine
   b. Levetiracetam
   c. Gabapentin
   d. Pregabalin
   e. Topiramate

Chapter 20 – Opioids - the basics and use in perioperative pain care

1. **Appropriate contexts for the use of opioid analgesia such as morphine include the following except (chose one or more):**
   a. Severe, nociceptive, acute pain
   b. Chronic, life-limiting, advancing pain
   c. Temporary relief of any pain

d. Chronic pain due to persistent pain generator as part of comprehensive treatment

e. Relief of common pains in patients with SUD

2. Potential harms of opioids include the following except:

a. High cost

b. Severe constipation

c. Sedation

d. Respiratory suppression

e. Death

f. Societal impacts due to increased substance use disorder

3. The benefits of modern peri-operative pain control include the following except:

a. Streamlined single-agent analgesia

b. Faster entry into physical rehabilitation

c. Reduced hypothalamic pituitary axis-mediated stress

d. Lowered rates of venous thrombosis

Chapter 21 – Opioids – the details: equianalgesia and safe use

1. The following are correct about opioid utilization in the United States except:

a. Daily morphine doses in excess of 90 mg day^{-1} should be avoided

b. Opioid prescriptions in the United States peaked in 2011 and have since declined

c. Patients with terminal cancer are likely to experience poorly controlled pain

d. Physiologically, opioids show stable efficacy over months to years

2. Regarding basic principles of safe opioid use according to CDC and JC guidelines, the following are appropriate except:

a. Combine opioids with non-pharmacological treatments

b. Combine opioids with benzodiazepines

c. Test patients for compliance with treatment

d. Limit opioids to the lowest effective dose for the shortest feasible time

3. The following are properties of opioids except:

a. Equianalgesia

b. Tachyphylaxis

c. Tolerance

d. Prophylaxis

Chapter 22 – Opioids – advanced practice - alternative delivery: IV, PCA, epidural

1. Which of the following administration routes is appropriate for a patient being discharged home one day after leg surgery. The patient is opioid-naïve, eating well, and anticipated to require three more days of opioid analgesia:

a. Transdermal

b. Oral

c. Intranasal

d. Buccal

e. IV

2. Which of the following routes may be utilized with morphine:

a. Oral, subcutaneous, intrathecal, rectal, but not IV

b. Oral, subcutaneous, intrathecal, rectal, IV

c. Oral, subcutaneous, intrathecal, IV, but not rectal

d. Oral, intrathecal, rectal, IV, but not subcutaneous

e. Oral, subcutaneous, rectal, IV, but not intrathecal

3. Which of the following is not an opioid with medical use in humans, per DEA:

a. Heroin

b. Methadone

c. Fentanyl

d. Morphine

e. Hydromorphone

Chapter 23 – Focal treatments for pain in primary practice: topical, iontophoretic, acupuncture, and basic injections

1. All of the following are focal treatments of pain, potentially administered or prescribed by primary care providers except:

a. OTC lidocaine cream

b. A fentanyl patch

c. Compounded neuropathy cream with amitriptyline, ketamine, and baclofen

d. Trigger point injections with saline

e. Selected local anesthetic blocks

2. The following agents are available for OTC use as topical pain-relieving agents, except:

a. Camphor

b. Ethanol

c. Salicylates

d. Capsaicin

e. Lidocaine

3. The following injections may be utilized in an office setting, given appropriate training except:

a. Greater occipital nerve blocks

b. Trigger point injections

c. Selected intra-articular steroid injections

d. Cervical epidural spinal injections

e. Botox injections

Chapter 24 – Interventional treatments and surgery for pain

1. Interventional and surgical treatments for radiating low back pain include the following except:

a. LESI

b. CESI

c. Spinal fusion

d. Medial branch block

e. Spinal cord stimulator

2. **Procedural techniques in general have**

a. High likelihood of success

b. Low likelihood of success

c. Variable likelihood of success, depending on technique and application

3. **The following best represents the time frame of relief most-typically provided by a Lumbar Epidural Steroid Injection (LESI):**

a. One day

b. Two weeks

c. Three months

d. Six months

e. One year

Chapter 25 – Activating therapies: PT, exercise, hydrotherapy, yoga and Chi Gong, sleep hygiene

1. **Activating therapies for pain include the following except:**

a. Yoga

b. Physical therapy

c. Massage

d. Meditation

e. Sleep tune-up

2. **Yoga has the following properties except:**

a. It can by maintained by patients after training

b. Consistent accomplishment of physical postures is the main focus

c. Some poses can make some pain conditions worse so training is needed

d. It can aid with balance, flexibility, and chronic pain

3. **Physical therapy features all of the following except:**

a. Musculoskeletal pain conditions often benefit from physical therapy

b. Physical therapy is typically associated with increased pain lasting five to seven days

c. Neuropathic pain conditions may benefit from skilled physical therapy

d. Physical therapies can apply a wide range of therapies including manual therapy, massage, iontophoresis, trigger point therapies, and stretching as well as exercise prescriptions and observed training

Chapter 26 – Mind-based therapies: CBT, ACT, reframing

1. **CBT includes the following main elements except:**

a. Commitment

b. Relaxation

c. Cognitive restructuring

d. Stress management

2. **Barriers to ACT include the following except:**

a. Lack of understanding of the method

b. Lack of evidence for efficacy

c. Lack of practitioners in this modality

d. Lack of appropriate patients

3. **Errors in cognition contributing to pain perpetuation include the following except:**

a. Optimism

b. All-or-none thinking

c. Leaping to conclusions

d. Overgeneralization

e. Catastrophizing

Chapter 27 – Manual therapies

1. **Manual therapies include the following except:**

a. Trigger point massage

b. Chiropractic manipulation

c. Lumbar fusion

d. Daily stretching

e. Traction

2. **Trigger points are associated with all of the following except:**

a. Self-treatment with dedicated massage techniques

b. Surgical excision

c. High levels of inflammatory mediators expressed in the site

d. A palpable firm knot or taut band in muscle

e. Predictable referred pain patterns

3. **Acupressure massage techniques are associated with all of the following except:**

a. Relief of some forms of pain

b. Highly specific patterns of pressure applied to locations on the body

c. Using a handheld device to apply pre-specified amounts of pressure

d. A conceptual foundation rooted in acupuncture medicine

e. Potential relief of other symptoms such as anxiety and insomnia that can worsen pain

Chapter 28 – Therapies that utilize descending pain pathways: meditation, vocation, games, music, and others

1. **All of the following are self-directed therapies that utilize the descending pain modulation system, except:**

a. Meditation

b. Sleep optimization

c. Music

d. Distraction

e. Acupuncture

2. **Costs or side effects of therapies that engage descending pain modulation include the following except:**

a. Time investment is required

b. Effort to build new habits

c. Some out-of-pocket expenses

d. Impaired cognition

e. Reorganization of home or work environment

3. **The following are true about the efficacy of therapies engaging descending pain modulation, except:**

a. Video games may not be equally effective at reducing pain for all persons

b. Empathic engagement may not be equally effective at reducing pain for all persons

c. Sleep optimization is only possible if pain is well-enough controlled to permit sleep to occur

d. Vocational engagement is a mandatory part of all counseling for chronic pain

e. Getting patients to agree to a trial of mindfulness meditation may require application of the stages of change model and motivational interviewing techniques

Chapter 29 – Acute and chronic pain: the basics

1. **The following pairs reflect the relative prevalence of major pain mechanisms in acute vs. chronic pain:**

a. Neuropathic pain is more prevalent in acute pain

b. Nociceptive pain is less prevalent in chronic pain

c. Inflammatory pain is more prevalent in chronic pain

d. Inflammatory pain is less prevalent in acute pain

2. **Chronic pain mechanisms include**

a. Allodynia, meaning pain that matches the type of stimulus presented

b. Hyperalgesia, meaning increased pain in response to a painful stimulus

c. Pain catastrophizing, a psychological process that amplifies pain

d. Brain changes associated with dampening of social behaviors associated with acute pain

e. Decreased sleep quality, leading pain to be perpetuated and worsened

3. **Chronic pain is often defined a pain lasting more than three months, but this definition may need to be modified for tissues that have normally long repair times, examples of tissues:injury pairs with long repair times include the following except:**

a. Muscle: complete tear

b. Muscle: sprain

c. Tendon: tendonitis

d. Bone: dislocation with spontaneous recurrence

e. Vertebral disc: rupture

Chapter 30 – Surgical and procedural pain

1. **Enhanced recovery after surgery (ERAS) is a**

a. Hospital-based initiative to improve surgical recovery

b. An international collaborative to collect data, study, educate, and audit perioperative factors to improve recovery

c. A US-based program sponsored by the NIH to enhance recovery after surgery and improve access to rehabilitation centers

2. **Psychological support includes making the patient well informed about the expectations for the following except:**

a. Rapid mobilization after surgery

b. Pain control after surgery

c. Psychological rounds the morning after surgery

d. Specific criteria for discharge

3. **The most common surgical procedures, aside from those for maternal/neonatal care, are performed for conditions commonly associated with pain, these include the following except:**

a. Knee replacement

b. Hip surgeries

c. Spine fusion

d. Spinal laminectomy

e. Cataract removal

Chapter 31 – Musculoskeletal pain

1. **All of the following are medication: lethality pairs except:**

a. NSAIDs: older adult on anticoagulation experiencing GI bleeding

b. Acetaminophen: hepatotoxicity in patient with pre-existing hepatic impairment

c. Acetaminophen: renal failure in patient with pre-existing alcoholism

d. Opioids: respiratory failure when combined with benzodiazepines

e. Opioids: respiratory failure in patient with pre-existing pulmonary disease

2. **Which of the following is not an element of a pain self-management plan for someone with musculoskeletal-related pain:**

a. Moderate daily exercise (as adapted to capability)

b. Taking extra medication and calling PCP to advocate for early refills

c. Sufficient restful sleep

d. Meditation or deep breathing

e. Thermal therapies: warm heating pad or cool pack

3. **Which of the following is not a consequence of musculoskeletal pain**

a. Decreased mood

b. Mild impairment in normal cognitive abilities

c. Focal muscle loss

d. Increased risk of falling

e. Prolonged sleep periods

Chapter 32 – Orofacial pain

1. **Pulpitis primarily arises from the following pain mechanisms:**

a. Nociceptive

b. Inflammatory

c. Neuropathic

d. Nociceptive and Inflammatory

e. Inflammatory and Neuropathic

2. **Trigeminal neuralgia presents with neuropathic pain of which cranial nerve:**

a. CN I (cranial nerve 1)

b. CN II

c. CN III

d. CN IV

e. CN V

3. **Temporomandibular joint disorder is managed with**

a. Carbamazepine

b. Comprehensive treatment

c. Liquid diet to avoid chewing

d. Vocal rest

e. Topical lidocaine

Chapter 33 – Neck pain, cervical and thoracic spine pain

1. **Cervical epidural steroid injection is more hazardous than lumbar epidural steroid injections because cervical spinal nerve roots are**

a. Shorter and more horizontally oriented than lumbar nerve roots

b. Shorter and more vertically oriented than lumbar nerve roots

c. Longer and more horizontally oriented than lumbar nerve roots

d. Shorter and more vertically oriented than lumbar nerve roots

2. **Cervical whiplash is**

a. Not a real syndrome

b. A syndrome with outcomes determined largely by psychological factors including depression, rumination, and worry

c. A syndrome with outcome determined by multiple factors including initially severe pain and injury mechanism

d. A syndrome that resolves quickly and leads to little disability

3. **Regarding facet joint osteoarthritis, the following are true except:**

a. Limits back bending (extension) of the cervical pain

b. Can result in pain that is both acute and chronic as well as dull and aching

c. Does not lead to neuropathic pain as nerve roots are not nearby

d. Responds to comprehensive management

e. May require the patient to participate actively in PT with a home exercise program for optimal results

Chapter 34 – Arm and hand pain

1. **Nerve compression syndromes producing pain in the arm and hand include all of the following except:**

a. Ulnar neuropathy at the lateral elbow

b. Carpal tunnel syndrome

c. "Saturday night palsy" of the radial nerve

d. C2 radiculopathy

e. Thoracic outlet syndrome

2. **Osteoarthritis is most common in the**

a. Shoulder

b. Elbow

c. Wrist

d. Hand

3. **Painful muscle tears are most common in the:**

a. Shoulder (supraspinatus muscle)

b. Forearm, e.g. extensor carpi ulnaris

c. Thumb base (abductor pollicus brevis)

d. Arm proper, e.g. triceps muscle

Chapter 35 – Low back pain: basic diagnosis and treatment planning

1. **The most important clue for diagnosing specific low back conditions associated with low back pain (excluding "red flag" diagnoses) is:**

a. Qualitative features of the pain, e.g. burning

b. Region, e.g. location in the back

c. Timing, e.g. occurs at night

d. Waxing and waning

e. Limitation in activity

2. **Sacroiliac joint pain is associated with the following except:**

a. Exquisite pain with movement

b. Localization to the low lateral back

c. Very focal (localizable) pain

d. Excellent response to oral analgesia

e. Partial relief with rest

3. **Disc degeneration is characterized by all the following except:**

a. Pain that is most often observed in young adults

b. Pain that is centrally located along the spine

c. Pain that occurs following cycles of inadequate conditioning and excessive strain

d. Pain that becomes much more intense when the disc is under pressure, e.g. sit-to-stand, sitting

e. Pain that often requires weeks-to-months to resolve each episode

Chapter 36 – Back pain emergencies

1. **Back pain emergencies include the following except:**

a. Vertebral fracture

b. Epidural abscess

c. Multifidus syndrome

d. Conus medullaris syndrome

e. Guillain–Barre syndrome

2. **MRI imaging is the preferred form of testing for the following except:**
   a. Spinal metastases
   b. Epidural abscess
   c. Conus medullaris syndrome
   d. Guillain–Barre syndrome
   e. Cauda equina syndrome
3. **The following are true about spinal metastases except:**
   a. Spinal metastases are common in patients with cancer at autopsy
   b. Spinal metastases are often associated with prostate and breast cancer
   c. Spinal metastases carry grave prognostic significance
   d. Spinal metastases do not produce much functional impairment
   e. Spinal metastases are treated with multiple therapeutic approaches

Chapter 37 – Radiating leg, buttock, and groin pain

1. **All of the following radiculopathies are common except:**
   a. L2
   b. L3
   c. L4
   d. L5
   e. S1
2. **Potential causes of meralgia paresthetica include the following except:**
   a. Obesity
   b. Herniated lumbar disc
   c. Pregnancy
   d. Tight belt-wearing
3. **Piriformis syndrome – which of the following is correct about treatment needs:**
   a. NSAIDs are needed
   b. Opioids are needed
   c. PT is needed
   d. Meditation is needed
   e. Seated rest is needed

Chapter 38 – Knee pain

1. **The following are major ligaments of the knee except:**
   a. Anterior collateral ligament
   b. Medial collateral ligament
   c. Anterior cruciate ligament
2. **The following are correct pairings of injury mechanism and injured knee structure:**
   a. ACL: knee hyperextension, change in direction with pivot
   b. PCL: fall onto flexed knee
   c. Meniscus: rapid change from forward to backward direction

   d. MCL: blow to lateral knee
   e. Iliotibial band: repeated running movement
3. **RICE-M acute care for sprain or strain includes the following except:**
   a. R: return to activity in 24 hours
   b. I: icing, cooling
   c. C: compression
   d. E: elevation
   e. M: medication

Chapter 39 – Foot and ankle pain

1. **The tarsal tunnel is located in the:**
   a. Lateral ankle
   b. Medial ankle
   c. Forefoot
   d. Plantar foot (inferior surface)
2. **Regarding Morton's neuroma, the following is true except:**
   a. Pain may be responsive to a gabapentinoid or podiatric treatment
   b. Lateral foot pressure or tight shoes may provoke shooting pain
   c. The nerve damage arises from chronic foot trauma
   d. Rapid referral is critical to treat this malignant tumor
3. **The population most likely to experience ankle sprain is**
   a. Teens
   b. Younger adults
   c. Middle-aged adults
   d. Older adults

Chapter 40 – Headache emergencies

1. **The following support diagnosis of subarachnoid hemorrhage except:**
   a. Indolent headache onset
   b. Changes in level of alertness
   c. Blood present in cerebrospinal fluid
   d. Imaging finding of blood surrounding intracranial skull-base structures
2. **The following contribute to the diagnosis of temporal arteritis except:**
   a. Older age
   b. Recent loss of sense of smell
   c. Elevated ESR (sedimentation rate)
   d. Systemic symptoms of weight loss, diffuse proximal pains, jaw claudication
   e. Temporal artery biopsy positive for vasculitis
3. **The following pairs are correct regarding meningitis and encephalitis except:**
   a. Meningitis: fever
   b. Encephalitis: seizure, focal neurological deficits

c. Meningitis: rapid administration of broad-spectrum antibiotics

d. Encephalitis: many CSF eosinophils

e. Encephalitis: may need additional CSF sample for virological testing

Chapter 41 – Headaches: basic diagnosis and management

1. **The following are characteristic of Tension type headache (TTH) except:**
   a. Throbbing hemicrania
   b. Worsening over course of the day
   c. Moderate severity
   d. Responds to NSAIDs or acetaminophen
   e. Patient self-manages the pain

2. **The following are characteristic of migraine except:**
   a. Photo- and phono-phobia
   b. Less common in women
   c. Responds to OTC analgesia, only if started within first few minutes of headache
   d. Disabling in severity
   e. Worsens with activity

3. **Headache diary is potentially all of the following except:**
   a. A tool for patient and provider to communicate about headache features like severity and timing
   b. Includes medications used for headache relief and changes to standing medications
   c. Can note changes in diet, exposure to headache triggers, or special activities
   d. A minute-to-minute log of the headache pain experience for a sample headache
   e. Can include documentation for multiple different headache types

Chapter 42 – Chronic headaches

1. **The following are true of chronic headaches except:**
   a. Chronic headaches may be intermittent
   b. Chronic headaches may wax and wane in intensity and pain may be absent at times
   c. Chronic headaches are not associated with more typical, acute headaches
   d. Chronic headaches often interfere with work and school productivity
   e. Chronic headaches are appropriate for comprehensive management

2. **About chronic migraine headache, the following are true except:**
   a. Chronic migraine headache typically occurs in isolation from other headaches
   b. Chronic migraine headache may present with bilateral headache
   c. Chronic migraine headache may present daily head pain

d. Chronic migraine headache may respond to comprehensive management

e. Chronic migraine headache may require daily preventative (prophylactic) medication

3. **The following is true about comprehensive management of headache except:**
   a. Psychological factors have a substantive role in improving chronic headaches
   b. Physical activity should be avoided in the management of chronic headache
   c. Ergonomic adaptation is important in managing chronic headaches
   d. Making sure that sleep is sufficient and not perturbed by conditions such as obstructive sleep apnea is appropriate
   e. Medications are an important part of comprehensive management of chronic headache

Chapter 43 – Visceral pain

1. **The following are considered chronic visceral pain syndromes except:**
   a. Inguinal hernia
   b. IBS (inflammatory bowel syndrome)
   c. Interstitial cystitis
   d. Chronic pancreatitis
   e. Esophagitis

2. **The following are distinctive features of visceral pain compared with somatic pain:**
   a. Signaling with neurotransmitters commonly identified as nociceptive
   b. Signaling with visceral-specific neurotransmitters
   c. Referred pain
   d. Colicky pain, i.e. pain in waves
   e. Distinct localization of pain

3. **Atypical cardiac pain is characterized by the following except:**
   a. Lower mortality
   b. Female preponderance
   c. Radiation into the left arm
   d. Description as discomfort
   e. Association with family history of MI

Chapter 44 – Pelvic pain

1. **Which of the following is the most prevalent conditions associated with pelvic pain in women?**
   a. Endometriosis
   b. Vaginismus
   c. Pelvic muscle trigger points
   d. Dysmenorrhea
   e. Pelvic congestion syndrome

2. **Which of the following is not a musculoskeletal pain condition of the pelvis?**

a. Prostadynia
b. Levator anus trigger points
c. Sacroiliac joint dysfunction
d. Symphysis pubis osteoarthritis
e. Hip osteoarthritis

3. **Which of the following pairs is not correct?**
   a. Sacroiliac joint dysfunction: both genders
   b. Coccydynia: male gender
   c. Endometriosis: female gender
   d. Dysmenorrhea: female gender
   e. Testicular pain: male gender

Chapter 45 – Exceptional causes of severe, chronic pain: CRPS, fibromyalgia, erythromelalgia, and small fiber peripheral neuropathy

1. **Which, among the exceptional causes of pain, is a not uncommon condition?**
   a. Small fiber peripheral neuropathy
   b. Fabry disease
   c. Erythromelalgia
   d. CRPS

2. **Fibromyalgia is characterized by the following non-pain symptoms, except:**
   a. Fatigue
   b. Intermittent rash
   c. Sleep disturbance
   d. Difficulty concentrating

3. **Which of the following is an incorrect pattern of pain cause with pain pattern:**
   a. Small fiber peripheral neuropathy: both feet initially worsening to involve both legs and hands
   b. Erythromelalgia: both feet initially worsening to involve both legs and hands
   c. Fibromyalgia: widespread and multifocal pain
   d. CRPS: pain involving one half of the body, i.e. hemi-body pain

Chapter 46 – Management of pain with substance abuse

1. **Patients in opioid withdrawal exhibit the following except:**
   a. Anxiety
   b. Pupil dilation
   c. Piloerector response
   d. Increased resistance to spontaneous and provoked pain
   e. Diarrhea

2. **Patients with chronic pain and substance use disorders benefit from comprehensive management strategies that include the following except:**
   a. Abrupt discontinuation of pharmacological treatments
   b. Psychological support
   c. Sleep hygiene

d. Moderate daily exercise
e. Avoidance of stress

3. **The following is correct about patients with chronic opioid exposure except:**
   a. These patients exhibit lower pain thresholds and lower pain tolerance
   b. Opioids become less effective in producing analgesia over time
   c. Non-pharmacological therapies are much more effective against pain in these patients
   d. Opioids continue to produce problematic side effects such as respiratory suppression

Chapter 47 – Pain at the end of life, opioid rotation

1. **The following are symptoms that may be associated with end-of-life except:**
   a. Pain
   b. Confusion
   c. Anxiety
   d. Agility
   e. Dyspnea

2. **The following represent elements of the hierarchy of needs, except:**
   a. Safety
   b. Physiology
   c. Self-realization or self-actualization
   d. Resolution
   e. Personhood (dignity)
   f. Socio-emotional

3. **The following are needs that can be identified as present in all phases of palliative care except:**
   a. Symptom management
   b. Spiritual or secular needs for meaning
   c. Psychosocial support
   d. Definitive cure

Chapter 48 – Opioids for chronic pain: preventing iatrogenic opioid use disorders

1. **The following are identified in this chapter as steps to prevent iatrogenic opioid use disorder:**
   a. Avoid escalating opioids
   b. Utilize opioids as part of a comprehensive pain management plan
   c. Only prescribe opioids to patients who have been interviewed and examined directly and for whom a differential diagnosis has been developed, with a diagnosis appropriate for opioid management as a lead diagnosis
   d. Check and document findings of a PDMP (Prescription Data Monitoring Program) prior to prescribing

e. Encourage staff to tell patients that all pain can be completely controlled

2. **The following standards have contributed to current practice standards regarding opioid prescribing, except:**
   a. Requirement for 40 hours of advanced practice training for physicians to qualify for Drug Enforcement Agency (DEA) controlled substance prescribing license
   b. Publication of universal precautions for prescribing opioids
   c. Creation of Prescription Data Monitoring Programs (PDMP) in essentially all states in the United States
   d. Release and dissemination of prescribing guidelines by the Centers for Disease Control

3. **The following are healthcare factors with potential to increase harms of opioids except:**
   a. Chronic respiratory disease
   b. Concurrent central nervous system (CNS) depressant medications
   c. High conscientiousness on personality testing
   d. Pre-existing opioid use disorder
   e. Suicidality

Chapter 49 – Tapering opioids in patients with pain

1. **The following are symptoms of opioid overdose except:**
   a. Agitation
   b. Myosis (pinpoint pupils)
   c. Constipation
   d. Suppressed or absent breathing
   e. Hypotension

2. **The following are symptoms of opioid withdrawal, except:**
   a. Cool dry skin
   b. Lacrimation
   c. Diarrhea
   d. Hypertension
   e. Chills and aches

3. **The following are correct about naloxone administration except:**
   a. Effects can wear off quickly
   b. Respiratory support may be needed for an extended period
   c. Patients may be found unconscious in hazardous settings – assessment is needed
   d. Patients will experience a profound sense of relief with administration
   e. Naloxone can be formulated for intranasal or intramuscular administration

Chapter 50 – Pain in infants, children, and adolescents

1. **Common techniques recommended for relieving pain in infants include the following except:**
   a. Video watching
   b. Soft music or singing to the infant
   c. Gentle holding while seating in a rocking chair
   d. Wrapping or swaddling as instructed
   e. Gentle touch or soothing stroking

2. **The following correctly match pediatric pain to pain scale except:**
   a. Neonate: NIPS
   b. Small child: FLACC
   c. Preadolescent, verbal: Wong-Baker
   d. Adolescent, nonverbal: NRS (numerical rating scale)

3. **Common causes of pain in adolescent and teen patients include all of the following except:**
   a. Athletic injuries: sprains, strains, fractures
   b. Repetitive use injuries
   c. Colic
   d. Headaches, including migraines

Chapter 51 – Pain in older adults

1. **The following are common pain conditions in older adults except:**
   a. Dysmenorrhea
   b. Low back pain
   c. Knee pain
   d. Hip pain
   e. Neck pain

2. **The following are adaptations for comprehensive pain management in older adults paired with an appropriate rationale except:**
   a. Ergonomic bathroom grab-bars: falls are an important cause of pain in older adults
   b. Gentle yoga or Qi gong: mind–body therapies are especially effective for chronic musculoskeletal pain
   c. Careful and monitored use of NSAIDs, potentially with gastroprotection: older adults have increased risk for GI bleeding
   d. Increased spinal injection of steroids: shortened lifespan means side effects are not relevant
   e. Acceptance Commitment Therapy for pain: older adults have potential for meaning-based therapy

3. **The following are appropriate medication strategies paired with prescribing rationales for older adults except:**
   a. Prescribe decreased NSAIDs due to risks for GI bleeding and vascular events
   b. Prescribe muscle relaxants frequently as older adults have a high rate of musculoskeletal pain
   c. Prescribe neuromodulating agents, such as gabapentinoid starting at low dose and tapering up slowly due to increased complications of baseline reduced balance and likelihood of wooziness as a side effect
   d. Prescribe pain-active antidepressants only after counseling about black box suicidality risks as older adults have increased risk for death by suicide
   e. Refer patients for interventional pain management as the side effect profiles may be beneficial relative to systemic medications

Chapter 52 – Tailoring pharmacotherapy in aging, renal, liver, and other metabolic dysfunction

1. **The following are correct pairs regarding medication: age-related changes impacting pharmacotherapy:**
   a. NSAIDs: high absolute rates of renal impairment mean prescreening is appropriate prior to use
   b. Acetaminophen: high absolute rates of hepatic impairment limit practical use
   c. Gabapentinoids: patients with increased fall risks should have medication started at a low dose with gradual dose adjustments
   d. Benzodiazepines: factors of increased adipose tissue, decreased lean body mass, increased cognitive impairment, and decreased gait stability increase potential harms
   e. Opioids: prevalence of respiratory impairments, including sleep apnea, increases associated risks for mortality

2. **Older adults have increased rates of the following conditions, increasing risks for analgesia, except:**
   a. Dementia
   b. Chronic respiratory disease
   c. Impaired gait of multifactorial origin
   d. Chronic renal failure
   e. Substance use disorders

3. **Renal failure means the following medications are contraindicated or strictly limited except:**
   a. Acetaminophen
   b. Ibuprofen
   c. Naproxen
   d. Gabapentin

Chapter 53 – Pain in pregnancy and the puerperium

1. **Which of the following is considered safe throughout pregnancy and lactation:**
   a. Acetaminophen
   b. Ibuprofen
   c. Oxycodone
   d. Valproic acid

2. **Which of the following time periods is ibuprofen contraindicated:**
   a. First trimester
   b. Second trimester
   c. Late pregnancy, i.e. after 30 weeks' gestation
   d. Breastfeeding

3. **Which of the following cannot be adapted for safe use during pregnancy:**
   a. Physical activity
   b. Psychological support
   c. High dose opioids
   d. Sleep hygiene
   e. Mind–body therapies

Answers

Chapter 1: 1. d, 2. d, 3. a

Chapter 2: 1. b, 2. c, 3. a

Chapter 3: 1. c, 2. b, 3. b

Chapter 4: 1. c, 2. d, 3. c

Chapter 5: 1. b, 2. c, 3. d

Chapter 6: 1. a, 2. b, 3. d

Chapter 7: 1. d, 2. c, 3. b

Chapter 8: 1. b, 2. d, 3. d

Chapter 9: 1. d, 2. c, 3. e

Chapter 10: 1. c, 2. a, 3. d

Chapter 11: 1. a, 2. e, 3. d

Chapter 12: 1. a, 2. d, 3. a

Chapter 13: 1. e, 2. b, 3. c

Chapter 14: 1. a, 2. e, 3. c

Chapter 15: 1. a, 2. a, 3. a

Chapter 16: 1. e, 2. d, 3. a

Chapter 17: 1. d, 2. d, 3. b

Chapter 18: 1. c, 2. d, 3. b

Chapter 19: 1. d, 2. a, 3. b

Chapter 20: 1. c, 2. a, 3. a

Chapter 21: 1. d, 2. b, 3. d

Chapter 22: 1. b, 2. b, 3. a

Chapter 23: 1. b, 2. b, 3. d

Chapter 24: 1. d, 2. c, 3. b

Chapter 25: 1. c, 2. b, 3. b

Chapter 26: 1. a, 2. b, 3. a

Chapter 27: 1. c, 2. b, 3. c

Chapter 28: 1. e, 2. d, 3. d

Chapter 29: 1. a, 2. a, 3. b

Chapter 30: 1. b, 2. c, 3. e

Chapter 31: 1. c, 2. b, 3. e

Chapter 32: 1. a, 2. e, 3. b

Chapter 33: 1. a, 2. c, 3. c

Chapter 34: 1. d, 2. d, 3. a

Chapter 35: 1. b, 2. d, 3. a

Chapter 36: 1. c, 2. d, 3. d

Chapter 37: 1. a, 2. b, 3. c

Chapter 38: 1. a, 2. c, 3. a

Chapter 39: 1. b, 2. d, 3. a

Chapter 40: 1. a, 2. b, 3. d

Chapter 41: 1. a, 2. b, 3. d

Chapter 42: 1. c, 2. a, 3. b

Chapter 43: 1. a, 2. e, 3. c

Chapter 44: 1. d, 2. a, 3. b

Chapter 45: 1. a, 2. b, 3. d

Chapter 46: 1. d, 2. a, 3. c

Chapter 47: 1. d, 2. d, 3. d

Chapter 48: 1. e, 2. a, 3. c

Chapter 49: 1. a, 2. a, 3. d

Chapter 50: 1. a, 2. b, 3. c

Chapter 51: 1. a, 2. d, 3. b

Chapter 52: 1. b, 2. e, 3. a

Chapter 53: 1. a, 2. c, 3. c

Index

Pain Medicine at a Glance, First Edition. Beth B. Hogans.
© 2022 John Wiley & Sons Ltd. Published 2022 by John Wiley & Sons Ltd.